Pediatric and Adolescent Gynecology

Pediatric and Adolescent Gynecology

A Problem-Based Approach

Edited by

Sarah M. Creighton
University College Hospital, London

Adam Balen
University of Leeds

Lesley Breech
Cincinnati Children's Hospital

Lih-Mei Liao
University College Hospital, London

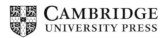
CAMBRIDGE
UNIVERSITY PRESS

CAMBRIDGE
UNIVERSITY PRESS

University Printing House, Cambridge CB2 8BS, United Kingdom

One Liberty Plaza, 20th Floor, New York, NY 10006, USA

477 Williamstown Road, Port Melbourne, VIC 3207, Australia

314–321, 3rd Floor, Plot 3, Splendor Forum, Jasola District Centre, New Delhi – 110025, India

79 Anson Road, #06–04/06, Singapore 079906

Cambridge University Press is part of the University of Cambridge.

It furthers the University's mission by disseminating knowledge in the pursuit of education, learning, and research at the highest international levels of excellence.

www.cambridge.org
Information on this title: www.cambridge.org/9781107165137
DOI: 10.1017/9781316691502

First published 2018

Printed in the United Kingdom by Clays, St Ives plc

A catalogue record for this publication is available from the British Library.

Library of Congress Cataloging-in-Publication Data
Names: Creighton, Sarah M., editor. | Balen, Adam H., editor. | Breech, Lesley, editor. | Liao, Lih-Mei, editor.
Title: Pediatric and adolescent gynecology : a problem-based approach / edited by Sarah M. Creighton, Adam Balen, Lesley Breech, Lih-Mei Liao.
Other titles: Pediatric and adolescent gynecology (Creighton)
Description: Cambridge, United Kingdom ; New York, NY : Cambridge University Press, 2017. | Includes bibliographical references.
Identifiers: LCCN 2017042534 | ISBN 9781107165137 (hardback)
Subjects: | MESH: Genital Diseases, Female | Adolescent | Child | Infant
Classification: LCC RJ478 | NLM WS 360 | DDC 618.100835–dc23
LC record available at https://lccn.loc.gov/2017042534

ISBN 978-1-107-16513-7 Hardback

Contents

Contributors

Julie Alderson BSc, MSc, DPsychol
University Hospitals Bristol, Bristol, UK

Dr Sveta Alladi MBBS, MA, MPH, MRCPCH
Specialist Registrar in Community Child Health Great Ormond Street Hospital, London

Lisa Allen MD, FRCPC
Section of Pediatric and Adolescent Gynecology, The Hospital for Sick Children, Toronto, Ontario, Canada

Leslie A. Appiah, MD
University of Kentucky College of Medicine Kentucky Children's Hospital, Department of Obstetrics and Gynecology

Thomas R. Aust MD, MRCOG
Department of Obstetrics and Gynecology, Wirral University Teaching Hospital, UK. Department of Pediatric Surgery, Alder Hey Children's Hospital, Liverpool, UK.

Adam Balen MD, DSc, FRCOG
The Leeds Centre for Reproductive Medicine, Seacroft Hospital, Leeds, UK

Lesley Breech MD
Division of Pediatric and Adolescent Gynecology, Cincinnati Children's Hospital, Cincinnati, OH, USA

Gail Busby MRCOG
St Mary's Hospital, Manchester, UK

Stefanie Cardamone MD
New York University School of Medicine, Department of Obstetrics and Gynecology, Pediatric and Adolescent Gynecology

Paul M. Chadwick
Health Psychology Research Group, University College London, London, UK

Gerard S. Conway MD, FRCP
Endocrine and Metabolic Unit, University College London Hospital, London, UK

Sarah M. Creighton MD, FRCOG
Department of Women's Health, University College Hospital, London

Naomi S. Crouch MD, MRCOG
Division of Obstetrics and Gynecology, University Hospitals Bristol, Bristol, UK

Alfred Cutner MD, FRCOG
Elizabeth Garrett Anderson and Obstetric Hospital, University College London Hospitals NHS Trust, London, UK

Melanie C. Davies MBBS, MRCP, FRCOG
University College London Hospitals and Institute of Women's Health, University College, London

Rebecca Deans PhD, FRANZCOG, CREI
UNSW Royal Hospital for Women, Randwick NSW, Australia

Jennifer E. Dietrich MD, MSc, FACOG
Department of Obstetrics and Gynecology and Department of Pediatrics, Baylor College of Medicine and Texas Children's Hospital

Margaret Hall-Craggs MRCP, FRCR, MD
Consultant Radiologist and Professor of Medical Imaging, UCL

Deborah Hodes MBBS, BSc, DRCOG, FRCPCH
University College London Hospitals NHS Foundation Trust, Camden Clinical Commissioning Group and Royal Free London NHS Foundation Trust

Anette Jacobsen BAO, LRCP&SI, FRCSI
KK Women's and Children's Hospital, Singapore

Davor Jurkovic MD, PhD, FRCOG
Department of Obstetrics and Gynecology,
University College London Hospital,
London, UK

Sari L. Kives MD
Department of Obstetrics and Gynecology,
University of Toronto, Toronto, Ontario,
Canada

Lih-Mei Liao PhD, MSc, FBPsS
Women's Health Division, University College
London Hospital, London, UK

Diane F. Merritt MD
Department of Obstetrics and Gynecology
Division of Pediatric and Adolescent Gynecology,
Washington University School of Medicine, St. Louis,
MO, USA

Lina Michala MRCOG, PhD
Division of Pediatric and Adolescent Gynecology,
First Department of Obstetrics and Gynecology,
University of Athens

Miriam Muscarella
University of California San Francisco School of
Medicine

Anne-Marie Amies Oelschlager MD
Department of Obstetrics and Gynecology, University
of Washington School of Medicine and Seattle
Children's Hospital

Katrina Roen PhD
Department of Psychology, University of Oslo, Oslo,
Norway

Anne Tamar-Mattis
interACT, Sudbury, Massachusetts, USA

Alun Williams MA, FRCS
Department of Pediatric Urology, University of
Nottingham Queen's Medical Centre, Nottingham, UK

Cara Williams MBChB, MRCOG
Liverpool Women's Hospital and Alder Hey
Children's Hospital, Liverpool

Dan Wood PhD, FRCS, FRCS (Urol)
University College London Hospital, London, UK

Paul L. Wood MD, FRCOG
Cambridge University Hospitals, Cambridge, UK

Michal Yaron MD
Department of Obstetrics and Gyneocology,
Department of Pediatric and adolescent, Pediatric
and adolescent gynecology; Geneva University
Hospitals, Geneva, Switzerland

Ephia Yasmin MD, MRCOG
Women's Health Division, University College
London Hospitals, London, UK

Jennie Yoost MD, MSc
Marshall University Department of Obstetrics and
Gynecology, Huntington, WV, USA

An Introduction to Pediatric and Adolescent Gynecology Practice

Adam Balen, Lesley Breech, Sarah M. Creighton, and Lih-Mei Liao

Introduction

Pediatric and adolescent gynecology (PAG) is now a recognized subspecialty that encompasses a spectrum of conditions affecting gynecological health from birth through to adulthood. Serious and life-threatening diseases may be relatively rare, but problems such as atypical development of the genital tract are highly complex. The development of specialist centers is important for appropriate and timely referral. For conditions that affect fertility, sexuality, health, and well-being, multidisciplinary care is the gold standard. In addition, for conditions requiring lifelong care, the development of methodical transition from pediatric to adolescent and adult services is necessary. Collaborative clinical networks not only promote quality and consistency in care delivery, they also improve professional learning and raise the standard of research.

History of PAG

Until relatively recently girls with gynecological conditions – particularly when surgery was required – were managed by adult general gynecologists and general surgeons [1,2]. This began to change more than 75 years ago with the opening of the world's first clinic for children with gynecological problems in Prague in 1940. The work of Professor Sir Jack Dewhurst from the 1960s onward recognized the need for specialist dedicated clinics and collaborative working between health care professionals. Schauffler published the first textbook on pediatric gynecology in 1947 [3]; this was followed by other textbooks, manuals, and atlases published from around the world including texts by Dewhurst in 1963 and 1980 [4,5], Huffman in 1968 [6], and Emans in 1977 [7]. The *Journal of Adolescent and Pediatric Gynecology* was first published in 1987.

As for all branches of medicine, investigation and treatment should be underpinned by scientific advances. The understanding of pubertal growth and development guided by the definitions by Marshall and Tanner for breast and pubic hair development and growth velocity [8] has enabled conditions to be more clearly described. Improvement of survival rates of childhood conditions has resulted in many more children born with complex medical conditions becoming young adults with sexual and reproductive aspirations. Environmental and societal factors have influenced the prevalence of sexual risk taking, substance misuse, smoking, and obesity, all of which can impact the general and gynecological health of adolescents and young women. Advances in gynecological investigation and treatments include imaging and minimal access surgery as well as hormonal interventions and the introduction of the contraceptive pill. These have dramatically expanded treatment options and choices for girls and young women.

Whereas earlier descriptions in the medical literature focused primarily upon descriptions of surgical techniques for congenital anomalies [9], more recent publications highlight the transition of PAG to a clearly defined subspecialty requiring specific knowledge and surgical as well as nonsurgical clinical skills. In the context of these developments, a number of clinical and scientific networks have emerged to encourage research and provide education and training (Table 1.1). National and international organizations launched include BritSPAG (the British Society for Pediatric and Adolescent Gynecology), ALOGIA (Asociación Latinoamericana de Obstetrica y Ginecologia Infantil y de la Adolescente), FIGIJ (Federation Internationale de Gynecologic Infantile et Juvenile), NASPAG (North American Society for Pediatric and Adolescent Gynecology), and most recently EUROPAG (European Association of Pediatric and Adolescent Gynecology). An important brief of these organizations is to facilitate the development of comprehensive and high-quality clinical services whereby children are appropriately

Table 1.1 Milestones in the Development of the Specialty of Pediatric and Adolescent Gynecology

Year	Event
1940	Professor Rudolf Peter Prague, Czech Republic Opening of world's first dedicated clinic for pediatric gynecology
1947	Publication of "Pediatric Gynecology" by Dr. Goodrich Shaffer
1963	Professor Sir J. Dewhurst published "The Gynaecological Disorders of Infants and Children."
1971	FIGIJ Federation Internationale de Gynecologic Infantile et Juvenile
1986	NASPAG North American Society for Pediatric and Adolescent Gynecology
1987	First issue of *Journal for Pediatric and Adolescent Gynecology*
1993	ALOGIA Asociación Latinoamericana de Obstetrica y Ginecologia Infantil y de la Adolescente
1997	International Fellowship of Pediatric and Adolescent Gynecology
2000	BritSPAG British Society for Pediatric and Adolescent Gynecology
2008	EUROPAG European Association of Pediatric and Adolescent Gynecology

referred and data usefully collected. A collective aspiration that must keep going is to take courageous and collective steps to tackle global health inequalities in PAG [10].

Pediatric and Adolescent Gynecological Conditions

Puberty is typically characterized by a series of biomarkers between the ages of 10 and 16. Although the precise mechanisms that regulate physical growth and pubertal onset are still not clearly understood, they are known to be influenced by a multitude of factors including genetic, social, economic, health, and lifestyle conditions. While changes are usually gradual, menarche is a discreet event that can be dated in girls, whose reproductive and sexual maturity may not be matched by their cognitive and emotional development. Clinical management must also take into account the overall developmental trajectory of the adolescent girl and the familial and social contexts.

The type of conditions treated by PAG specialists can be expected to vary to some extent across regions and nations. In the United States, for example, teenage sexual health is an important part of the remit, whereas in the United Kingdom, this is provided by nationally organized sexual health clinics within a community setting rather than in an acute hospital service. Menstrual disorders make up a large proportion of work in most PAG clinics. Polycystic ovary syndrome (PCOS) and prepubertal vulval dermatological complaints are also common. Most cases of abnormal uterine bleeding in adolescence are due to anovulatory cycles during the first 12 to 18 months after menarche, which is related to underdevelopment of the hypothalamic-pituitary-ovarian axis. Menorrhagia may be related to a bleeding diathesis and occasionally to systemic illness or structural lesions. The principles of investigation are the same as for adult women and can be initiated in the primary sector. Even so, referrals to specialist PAG clinics have increased [11], reflecting perhaps a reluctance among general practitioners and general gynecologists to manage relatively straightforward conditions without specialist input.

Other conditions treated in PAG services include disorders of pubertal development. Primary and secondary amenorrhea and precocious puberty may be associated with complex underlying conditions and are best managed together with pediatric endocrinologists with access to developmental psychological input. Rokitansky Syndrome (müllerian agenesis, Mayer-Rokitnsky-Kuster-Hauser Syndrome, MRKH) is more common than perhaps realized with an incidence in the region of 1:5000 [12]. Ovarian function is unaffected and presentation is usually at adolescence. Primary amenorrhea is reported in the presence of typical secondary sex characteristics. The recent breakthrough of live uterine transplantation has attracted significant attention [13], although debates on ethics and health economics have yet to be advanced.

Complex congenital conditions associated with atypical development of chromosomal, gonadal, and anatomical sex are referred to as "disorders of sexual development" (DSD) [14]. Other preferred terms for this group of conditions include "differences in sex development" and "intersex." A DSD diagnosis may be made at any age and may include other body differences or physical health problems. Where the external genitalia appear atypical, the diagnosis of the underlying condition is often made in infancy. When the external genitalia look typical but the internal genitalia are not (e.g., absent or small vagina and/or uterus, presence of testes in a girl), the underlying condition may not be identified until adolescence following investigations for primary amenorrhea or virilization at puberty. Medical management of DSD is challenging and continues to evolve. Clinical care must be within a specialist multidisciplinary team with integrated psychological input. Surgery to "normalize" the genitals was accepted as routine in the past. The practice on children has been the focus of debate for the past two decades. Currently, it is framed as a breach of human rights [15]. Prophylactic gonadectomy, which must be followed by steroid replacement, is also under debate [16].

Cloacal anomalies are the most complex in the spectrum of anorectal malformations affecting 1 in 50,000 live births [17]. Diagnosed during pregnancy or at birth, they will initially be under the care of the pediatric surgical team. They encompass a wide array of complicated defects and pose a formidable technical challenge to surgeons. Gynecological input is required at the onset of puberty and multidisciplinary transition clinics are essential to enable young women to move from pediatric to adult care. Other developing fields include preservation of reproductive potential in girls treated for cancer in childhood or adolescence; this falls under the remit of PAG in some services.

Emergent and related global concerns affecting girls and women are female genital mutilation/cutting. Health issues in girls related to female genital mutilation/cutting often fall within the workload of the PAG specialist. Female genital mutilation (FGM) is defined by the World Health Organization (WHO) as composed of various procedures that remove or damage the external female genital organs for non-medical reasons [18]. The majority of FGM is performed on children [19] with potentially long-term physical and psychological consequences. Migration of families from FGM-practicing countries means that FGM is now a global health concern [20]. All PAG specialists must be aware of the health impact and the legal status of FGM in their own countries and be able to identify and protect girls at risk.

Ironically, in more affluent nations, the number of healthy young women accessing female genital cosmetic surgery (FGCS) is on the rise [21]. The claims to clinical needs for such interventions are dubious [22]. Research in the area is poor and partisan and the benefits are unclear [23,24]. Despite these reservations, bold claims are found in web advertisements that directly target consumers [25,26]. An Australian analysis of provider information has identified surgery as embedded in a neoliberal discourse of individual choice, self-improvement, and objectification. It stresses the rhetoric of choice, empowerment, and agency, thus creating an ideological foundation and justification for cosmetic surgery [27]. Global professional concerns are reflected in a series of position statements and ethical guidance [28,29]. The demarcation between FGM and FGCS is controversial and a recent committee opinion in May 2016 from the American College of Obstetricians and Gynecologists on breast and labial surgery in adolescents prompted widespread condemnation and a large online petition to withdraw the guidance [30]. There is a need to enhance education provided in schools about normal development during puberty and all aspects of sexual and reproductive health. In most countries sex and relationship education is variable, inconsistent, and inadequate.

Standards in PAG

Significant variability in PAG service provision across nations can be expected, as for other medical fields. Even within a country, variation may exist between different regions. In the UK, it is recognized that all acute hospitals should have a PAG lead clinician for children and adolescents with gynecological problems although not all hospitals will undertake management of complex PAG conditions. Although variations in service provision across national and international boundaries are inevitable, it is appropriate to aspire to core standards listed in Table 1.2.

It is recognized that adolescents with medical problems have special needs. Adolescents with gynecological problems have additional needs for privacy and sensitive handling. Many of the gynecological problems encountered relate to intimate bodily functions at a time when the individual is maturing sexually and having to deal with issues that are embarrassing and may be considered taboo. It is crucial to be aware of potential ethnic and cultural differences and communication challenges. For some families, it is often the father and not the mother who can speak English.

Table 1.2 Clinical Standards for Service Planning in PAG

Care needs to be in an appropriate setting with facilities for outpatient and inpatient management of children, adolescents, and their families.

There should be a designated lead clinician within each unit.

Children with gynecological problems should not be seen in the setting of an adult gynecology clinic.

All health care professionals involved in the management of these PAG cases should have completed appropriate training in safeguarding/child protection.

Clinical networks should be developed flexibly on a geographical basis to allow the transfer of care of complex cases from secondary/general PAG care to specialist centers.

There should be a limited number of designated specialist centers for the management of the very rare and more complex conditions. Specialist centers need to provide a multidisciplinary approach to treatment.

Basic and advanced training in PAG should be available.

Centers should maintain a database of cases

There is a need for important information to be available in different languages and for professional interpreters to assist in consultations. In some situations the preferences of the adolescents may not be the same as the wishes of the parents. Laws governing confidentiality and consent for adolescents vary from country to country. PAG specialists must ensure they are conversant with the governances that apply to their own clinical practice.

The Multidisciplinary Team (MDT)

Effective interdisciplinary care is critical for the care of adolescents with complex medical and surgical conditions, as well as for adolescents and young women accessing safe and reliable reproductive health care including contraceptive management. Since for many practicing pediatricians, the wide array of options for hormonal contraception may lie outside their usual scope of practice; a working interdisciplinary collaboration with gynecological colleagues to offer expertise and guidance is beneficial. In the tertiary care setting, psychosocial specialists are additional care providers on whom adolescents and young adults and their families struggling with the overwhelming health care environment can draw.

Pediatric psychological research across disease contexts has identified high-level parental stress to be an important determinant in unhelpful coping strategies such as distancing, escaping, and avoidance [31]. Fathers are thought to be more likely than mothers to distance themselves [32]. Parental

stress is reduced by being adequately informed about the child's condition and any interventions, and by opportunities to speak to other parents who have lived through similar experiences [33]. High maternal health, high maternal support, low maternal worry, and child-perceived control are associated with positive psychological adjustment in the diagnosed child [34]. The research in a variety of pediatric contexts makes a strong case for sustained psychological input for parents in pediatric gynecological care.

The UK guidance on DSD recommends as a minimum standard a clinical team of endocrinologists, surgeons and/or urologists, clinical psychologists/psychiatrists, radiologists, neonatologists, and specialist nurses. In addition, links to a wider group of specialties including plastic surgery, clinical genetics, clinical ethics forums, as well as the social services should be established. Patients, parents, and families should be signposted to peer support networks and forums. A team is not a collection of experts. What many guidelines have fallen short of is recommendations for the core conditions that are required for effective team function. However, even with such recommendations, skillful teamwork does not happen by chance but requires team development processes to realize its full potential. Without investment in team development, an MDT may not deliver the intended benefits to patients as it incurs substantial costs [35].

Transitioning from Pediatric and Adolescent to Adult Care

Adolescence is characterized by enormous changes in self-consciousness, identity, and cognitive flexibility [36]. Recent research using magnetic resonance imaging (MRI) of the adolescent brain describes changes associated with risk-taking and sensation-seeking behavior [37,38]. As young patients become more acutely aware of their diagnosis and the potential implications for physical appearance, sexuality, fertility, and general health, a resistance to the health care systems may emerge and be maintained by emotional avoidance and risk taking. Therefore, as more and more young people with serious medical conditions are surviving into adulthood, planned transition should be a care quality indicator. Adolescents and young adults with a history of complex medical conditions and/or previous reconstructive surgery may have difficulty in finding a gynecological care provider with the knowledge, skills, and experience to manage the long-term reproductive health following pediatric interventions. Risk of menstrual obstruction and sexual difficulties and unknown obstetric prognosis are just a few of the challenges. However, planned transition to adult care is important even for the more common chronic gynecological conditions such as lichen sclerosus, early diagnosis of polycystic ovarian syndrome, and endometriosis. Dedicated adolescent clinics can have an important role in providing a seamless handover [39]. However, there is currently little information to help PAG teams design methodical transitions [40]. The inertia can increase the risk of the young person becoming lost in transition [41]. Fortunately, planned transition is further advanced in other fields and PAG clinicians can learn from examples of good practice in other specialties [42,43]. Central to all such programs is the individualized plan for each child to reflect the development stage reached. Age-appropriate information resources and development of a departmental transition policy template are also important. These have been demonstrated to significantly improve knowledge about the disease, satisfaction with the clinical care, and health-related quality of life. However, funding models for this work are patchy and wider development of such programs will not happen without organizational commitment and financial investment.

With preparation for a well-planned transition to a trusted partner from the adult care model or a specialist embedded in the collaborative team within the adult health care system, patients can avoid adverse reproductive health consequences. Despite recognition of the importance of multidisciplinary transition for patients from pediatric to adult care, however, very few programs incorporate the full spectrum of providers. The provision of gynecological care is a significant gap in most transition programs. Even in the care of anorectal malformations, where there is a well-established association of reproductive tract anomalies, few programs include a gynecologist. The available literature in the field of transition medicine is limited in regard to transition in gynecology. This may be related to the relatively recent development of the subspecialty or pediatric providers lack of recognition of the associated gynecologic concerns or the long-term reproductive consequences of many conditions. The literature available describes a high proportion of adolescents who become lost to follow-up during transition and no longer receive appropriate adult services [44]. This suggests that clinicians are failing to transition young people safely even for complex conditions such as disorders of sex development [45].

An increase in communication and acknowledgment of identified future needs can help mitigate the current substantial gap in transition pathway development. Until resources are leveraged to both pediatric and adult care teams, such dedicated services are unlikely to increase. Increased opportunities for communication and mutual learning between pediatric and adult providers are required for progress.

Training and Education

PAG incorporates a wide range of conditions requiring different specialist skills and resources, and appropriate training and continuing professional education are essential. All PAG clinicians should be able to diagnosis and manage common problems and identify and initiate initial investigations for uncommon and more complex conditions. However, not all PAG specialists should treat highly complex conditions. Referral on to other appropriate specialist centers may be required for conditions such as cloacal anomalies, pediatric gynecological malignancies, DSD, gynecological aspects of other complex childhood conditions, sexual abuse, gender identity issues, and pregnancy in children and adolescents.

The syllabus of training programmes should be comprehensive to ensure that PAG trainees gain wide experience. To optimize professional learning and practice, the design of the content and process of training should be informed and supported by clear pedagogic frameworks. PAG fellowships of 1 to 2 years are increasingly popular and allow a breadth of clinical experience to be gained.

The number of training programs has substantially increased over the past 10–15 years as evidenced by the growth in North America (increasing from 2 long-standing centers to currently more than 10). The inherent challenge for the field of pediatric and adolescent gynecology is the broad crossover of both medical and surgical concerns stimulating interest from both medically and surgically based trainees. With this rich diversity of conditions and management, established US programs have cooperated to develop consistent core training goals and objectives to standardize the exposure and experience across the United States. Exposure to evaluation

5

and management of more basic general PAG issues as well as more complex medical and surgical concerns is important to prepare providers to practice in a tertiary care setting. Recognition of the role of the PAG-trained specialist has increased over the past decade in the United States with both the American Board of Obstetrics and Gynecology and the American College of Obstetricians and Gynecologists focusing specialized training programs and possible certification for designation of one's practice as PAG. An increasing number of independent US pediatric institutions have created full-time gynecology positions to provide reliable, consistent service to the pediatric, adolescent, and young adults receiving care in the pediatric system.

Conclusion

The developing field of PAG is like an open book to be read and enjoyed. The progression from a practical need to a recognized subspecialty in Europe, North America, and the rest of the globe has allowed opportunities for care providers and researchers to reach new heights in health care innovations to meet new challenges being identified daily. With such an exciting growth, there is no doubt that a previously overlooked clinical population will benefit from better, broader care.

The aspiration to better care has led to the recognition of the importance of better research. National and international provider organizations have encouraged multicenter PAG research collaborations by providing grant support. National funding in the areas of patient- and family-centered care for conditions affecting pediatric and adolescent gynecology such as disorders of sexual development, fertility preservation, and innovations in contraception have led to increased collaboration and focus on relevant research questions. Investigations in care quality improvement using tried and tested methodology have provided a framework to define the best model for the delivery of PAG care, permitting standardization of care to improve clinical outcomes in the long term.

References

1. McIndoe AH, Bannister JB An operation for the cure of congenital absence of the vagina. *J Obstet Gynaecol Br Emp* 1938; **45**: 490–494.

2. Davydov SN, Zhvitiascvili OD Formation of vagina (colpopoeisis) from peritoneum of Douglas pouch. *Acta Chir Plast* 1974; **16**(1): 35–41.

3. Shauffler GC *Pediatric Gynecology* 1947 Year Book Pub.

4. Dewhurst CJ *Gynaecological Disorders of Infants and Children* 1963 FA Davis.

5. Dewhurst CJ, Chamberlain G *Practical Pediatric and Adolescent Gynecology* 1980 Marcel Dekker.

6. Huffman JW *The Gynecology of Childhood and Adolescence* 1981 Saunders.

7. Emans SJ *Pediatric and Adolescent Gynecology* 1977 Little, Brown.

8. Marshall WA, Tanner JM Variations in pattern of pubertal changes in girls. *Arch Dis Child*. 1969; **44** (235): 291–303.

9. Yordan EE, Yordan RA The early historic roots of pediatric and adolescent gynecology. *J. Pediatr. Adolesc.Gynecol* 1997; **10**: 183–191.

10. Marmot M *The Health Gap: The Challenge of an Unequal World* 2015 Bloomsbury Publishing.

11. Kulkarni MA, Glanville JM, Phillott S et al. A review of Pediatric and Adolescent gynecology services in a tertiary outpatient clinic. *Human Fertility* 2017; **20**(3): 168–178.

12. Aittomäki KI, Eroila H, Kajanoja P A population-based study of the incidence of Müllerian aplasia in Finland. *Fert. Ster.* 2001; **76**(3): 624–625.

13. Brännström M, Johannesson L, Bokström H et al. Live birth after uterus transplantation *The Lancet* 2015; **385**: 607–616.

14. Lee PA, Nordenstrom A, Houk CP et al. and the Global DSD Update Consortium. Global disorders of sex development update since 2006: perceptions, approach and care. *Hormone Research in Pediatrics* 2016; **85**: 158–180.

15. Liao LM, Wood D, Creighton SM Parental choice on normalising cosmetic genital surgery. *BMJ* 2015 Sep 28.

16. Deans R, Creighton SM, Liao L-M et al. Timing of gonadectomy in adult women with complete androgen insensitivity syndrome: Patient preferences and clinical evidence. *Clinical Endocrinology* 2012, DOI: 10.1111/j.1365–2265.2012.04330.x.

17. Warne SA, Hiorns MP, Curry J et al. Understanding cloacal anomalies. *Archives of Disease in Childhood* 2011; **96**: 1072–1076.

18. World Health Organization (WHO). Female genital mutilation. Fact sheet No. 241, Updated Feb 2014 www.who.int/mediacentre/factsheets/fs241/en/.

19. UNICEF Female Genital Mutilation/Cutting: A statistical overview and exploration of the dynamics of change. July 2013 (www.unicef.org) www.unicef.org/media/files/FGCM_Lo_res.pdf.

20. Creighton SM, Dear J, de Campos C et al. Multidisciplinary approach to the management of

children with female genital mutilation (FGM) or suspected FGM: service description and case series. *BMJ Open.* 2016; **6**(2): e010311. DOI: 10.1136/bmjopen -2015–010311.

21. Liao LM, Creighton SM Requests for cosmetic genitoplasty: how should healthcare providers respond? *The British Medical Journal* 2007; **334**: 1090–1092.

22. Crouch NS, Dean R, Michala L et al. Clinical characteristics of women and girls seeking labia reduction surgery. *British Journal of Obstetrics & Gynecology* 2011. DOI: 10.1111/j1471-0528.2011.03088.

23. Braun V. Female genital cosmetic surgery: a critical review of current knowledge and contemporary debates. *J. Womens Health* 2010; **19**(7): 1393–1407.

24. Liao L-M, Michala L, Creighton S. Labial surgery for well women: a review of the literature. *British Journal of Obstetrics & Gynecology* 2010; **117**(1): 20–25.

25. Liao LM, Taghinejadi N, Creighton SM A content and implications analysis of online advertisements for female genital cosmetic surgery. *BMJ Open* 2012; **2**: e001908. DOI: 10.1136/bmjopen-2012–001908.

26. Tiefer L Female cosmetic genital surgery: freakish or inevitable. Analysis from medical marketing, bioethics and feminist theory. *Feminism Psychol.* 2008; **18**: 466–479.

27. Moran C, Lee C Selling genital cosmetic surgery to healthy women: a multimodal discourse analysis of Australian surgical websites. Critical Discourse Studies, 2013.

28. British Society for Pediatric & Adolescent Gynecology Position Statement Labial reduction surgery (Labiaplasty) on adolescents (2013). www .rcog.org.uk/ … /britspag_labiaplastypositionstate ment.pdf.

29. Royal College of Obstetricians and Gynaecologists Ethical opinion paper, Ethical considerations in relation to female genital cosmetic surgery (FGCS, 2013).

30. American College of Obstetrics and Gynecology Breast and Labial Surgery in Adolescents, Committee Opinion Number 662, May 2016.

31. Mednick L, Gargollo P, Oliva M et al. Stress and coping of parents of young children diagnosed with bladder exstrophy. *Journal of Urology* 2009; **181**: 1312–1317.

32. Azar R, Solomon CK Coping strategies of parents facing child diabetes mellitus. *Journal of Pediatric Nursing* 2001; **16**(6): 418–428.

33. Baratz A, Sharp MK, Sandberg DE Disorders of sex development Peer support. In: Hiort O, Ahmed SF (eds) *Understanding Differences and Disorders of Sex Development (DSD).* Endocr Dev. Basel, Karger 2014; **27**: 99–112 DOI: 10.1159/000363634.

34. Immelt S Psychological adjustment in young children with chronic medical conditions. *Journal of Pediatric Nursing* 2006; **31**(5): 362–377.

35. Ke KM, Blazeby JM, Strong S et al. Are multidisciplinary teams in secondary care cost-effective? A systematic review of the literature. *Cost Effectiveness and Resource Allocation* 2013; **11**: 7.

36. Rutter M, Rutter M *Developing Minds.* London: Penguin, 1993.

37. Goddings A-L, Mills K, Clasen L et al. Longitudinal MRI to assess effect of puberty on subcortical brain development: an observational study. *Lancet* 2014; **383**: 52.

38. Fuhrmann, D, Knoll, LJ, Blakemore, SJ Adolescence as a Sensitive Period of Brain Development. *Trends in Cognitive Sciences* 2015; **19**(10): 558–566. DOI:10.1016/j.tics.2015.07.008

39. McGreal S, Wood PL A study of peadiatric and adolescent gynecology services in a British district general hospital. *BJOG: An International Journal of Obstetrics and Gynecology* 2010; **117**: 1643–1650.

40. Liao L-M, Tacconelli E, Wood D et al. Adolescent girls with disorders of sex development: a needs analysis of transitional care. *Journal of Pediatric Urology* 2010; **6**: 609–613.

41. Viner RM Transition of care from pediatric to adult services; one part of improved health services for adolescents. *Arch Dis Child* 2001; **93**: 160–163.

42. Harden PN, Walsh G, Bandler N et al. Bridging the gap: an integrated pediatric to adult clinical service for young adults with kidney failure. *BMJ* 2012; **344**: e3718.

43. Nagra A, McGinnity PM, Davis N et al. Implementing transition: Ready Steady Go. *Arch Dis Child Edu Prac Ed* 2015; **100**: 313–320.

44. Gleeson H, Davis J, Jones J et al. The challenge of delivering endocrine care and successful transition to adult services in adolescents with congenital adrenal hyperplasia experience in a single centre over 18 years. *Clin. Endocrinol (Oxf)* 2013; **78**(1): 2308.

45. Gleeson H, Wisniewski AB Working with adolescents and young adults to support transition. *Endocr. Dev.* 2014; **27**: 128–137.

Chapter 2

Embryology and Normal Development of Female Reproductive Function in Pediatric and Adolescent Gynecological Practice

Cara Williams and Rebecca Deans

Development of the Gonads

Primordial germ cells originate from the primitive ecto-derm and, initially in their development, migrate out of the embryo into the yolk sac. By the 6th week, these primordial germ cells have migrated into the genital ridges of the intermediate mesoderm, multiplying by mitosis as they migrate. The genital ridges are located just ventromedial to the mesonephros. Somatic cells develop from the thickened coelomic epithelium of the genital ridge, and they surround and nourish the pri-mordial germ cells, forming gonadal cords. By the end of the 6th week, male and female gonads cannot be distinguished, and the gonad is sexually indifferent.

In the absence of a Y chromosome and lack of expression of the SRY gene, the mesonephric duct atro-phies and the gonadal cords degenerate. The germ cells differentiate into oogonia. The oogonia multiply by mitosis so that there are approximately 7 million by 20 weeks. They spontaneously enter the first phase of meio-sis and arrest in prophase where they are called the "primary oocytes." The granulosa cells develop out of the gonadal cord cells and surround the primary oocytes to form the primordial follicle. Steroidogenic theca cells develop in the surrounding ovarian stroma. There is progressive follicular atresia from the 16th week onward, resulting in approximately 2 million oocytes at birth. Germ cell development is then arrested until puberty.

The gubernaculum is an embryonic structure thought to connect the internal genital system to the inguinal abdominal wall in early fetal development. It is known that the male gubernaculum plays a role in the descent of the testicles into the scrotum; however, the role of the gubernaculum in females is less clear. In the absence of testosterone and anti-Mullerian hormone (AMH), the Mullerian ducts develop, inter-fering with the connection between the gubernaculum and the mesonephros and gonadal suspensory liga-ments. The gubernaculum grows over the Mullerian duct and the muscular fibers become incorporated into the Mullerian duct at the uterotubal junction, forming the origins of the round ligament. The caudal gonadal suspensory ligament becomes the ovarian sus-pensory ligament with the ovary descending, but only to the level of the pelvis [1].

Development of the Mullerian Ducts and External Genitalia

During the 6th week of development, two parameso-nephric (Mullerian) ducts develop just lateral to the mesonephric duct in both male and female embryos. In the absence of testosterone and AMH, the meso-nephric (Wollfian) ducts degenerate and the parame-sonephric (Mullerian) ducts continue to develop caudally and medially with midline fusion to create the fallopian tubes, uterus, cervix, and upper vagina.

The urogenital sinus forms by week 7. Cells prolifer-ate from the upper portion of the urogenital sinus to form structures called the "sinovaginal bulbs." These fuse to form the vaginal plate, which extends from the Mullerian ducts to the urogenital sinus. This plate begins to canalize, starting at the hymen and proceeding cra-nially to the cervix. This process is not complete until 21 weeks of gestation. The hymen remains intact until around 40 weeks, when it spontaneously ruptures to give a patent vagina.

The external genitalia consist of the genital tubercle, urogenital sinus, and the urethral and labioscrotal folds. In females, the genital tubercle becomes the clitoris, the urogenital sinus becomes the urethra and lower vagina, urethral folds develop into the labia minora, and the labioscrotal folds become the labia majora. External genitalia are recognizably female by week 12 of development.

Genetic Control of Sex Development

Sex development can be divided into two processes: sex differentiation, whereby the undifferentiated

Gonad development: Balance of opposing signals

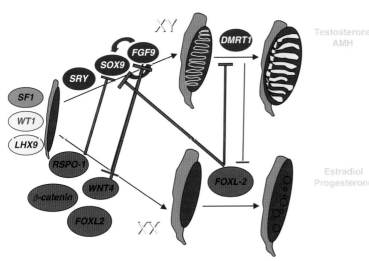

Figure 2.1 Gonad development: Balance of opposing signals [2].

gonad develops into either a testis or an ovary, and sex determination, whereby the phenotypic sex is determined based on what is produced by the differentiated gonad.

Genes involved in the development of the bipotential gonad have been identified, as knockout mice for these genes have been found to have complete absence of gonads. These include WT1 and LHX9, as well as NR5A1, which codes for steroidogenic factor 1 (SF1) [2].

The differentiation of the common gonadal primordium into an ovary is determined by a complex molecular interplay of pro-ovarian and anti-testis gene expression. In the gonadal ridge of the XX embryo, sexual dimorphism is triggered by R-spondin-1 (encoded by RSPO1) and FOXL2. WNT4, Fst, and β-catenin are also expressed, promoting development of the ovary. R-spondin-1 augments β-catenin signaling, possibly via WNT4 [3].

SF1 encodes a nuclear receptor that plays an important role in the development of the hypothalamic-pituitary-gonadal-adrenal axis. It is thought that SF1 is involved in the upregulation of SRY and SOX9 gene expression, two key testis-promoting genes [4]. DAX1 is a nuclear receptor protein that plays an important role in the development of the ovary. It is encoded by the NROB1 gene located on the short arm of the X chromosome. In mice models, over expression of DAX1 has been found to result in a reduction in the expression of SOX9, possibly via a direct inhibition of SF1-mediated transcription of the gene [5].

Activation of β-catenin signaling prevents SF-1 binding to TESCO in mice, thereby suppressing the male pathway. Additionally, R-spondin-1, FOXL2, WNT4, and β-catenin supress expression of SOX9 and FGF9 (another testis-promoting gene) and therefore prevent differentiation of testes. This antagonistic relationship between SOX9/FGF9 and the ovarian genes is mutual (Figure 2.1) [2,6].

Pathophysiology of Puberty

The onset of pubertal development is heralded by an increase in pulsatile release of GnRH from the hypothalamus. GnRH neurons are known to be mature from birth onward. Following brief activation in the neonatal period, they remain in a dormant state until the onset of puberty. The mechanism for this is thought to be a central inhibition independent of gonadal steroid feedback. The underlying cause of this central inhibition, however, is unclear. Estradiol levels in the stalk-median eminence of female rhesus macaques have been shown to be elevated in the prepubertal state with a subsequential drop in early puberty associated with an increase in GnRH pulsatility, suggesting a possible role for neurestradiol in the central inhibition of GnRH [7].

Pulsatile GnRH release causes gonadotropic cells of the anterior pituitary to release luteinizing hormone (LH) and follicle-stimulating hormone (FSH). LH stimulates production of Androstenedione in the ovarian theca cells, and FSH stimulates the synthesis

9

of estradiol in the granulosa cells under the influence of aromatase enzymes. The pulsatile release of GnRH begins before the onset of pubertal changes. Approximately one year prior to breast budding, pre-pubertal girls have elevated LH levels during sleep secondary to GnRH pulses. At the start of breast budding, LH and FSH peak amplitudes increase 10-fold and 2-fold, respectively. By Tanner stage 3, basal LH levels are usually detectable during the day. As puberty progresses, these peak amplitudes increase further and estradiol becomes detectable throughout the day. After approximately one year of daily estradiol production, menarche occurs, usually corresponding to the end of Tanner stage 4 [8].

Genetics of Puberty

Kisspeptins, encoded by the KISS1 gene, are a family of neuropeptides that causes activation of the G protein-coupled receptor 54 (GPR54). This receptor is co-localized to GnRH neurons in the arcuate nucleus of the hypothalamus. Kisspeptin signaling via the receptor is thought to play a part in initiating the GnRH pulse generator [9,10].

Neurokinin B (NKB) is a neurotransmitter peptide that is expressed in the same neurons that express kisspeptin. NKB is encoded for by the TAC3 gene, and its receptor NKR3 by TACR3. Mutations in TAC3 and TACR3 have been found to result in hypogonadism [11].

MKNR3 is another gene that has been linked to puberty. A loss of function of the MKNR3 gene has been found in familial cases of precocious puberty, suggesting that MKNR3 plays a role in inhibiting puberty. However, the exact mechanism for this is unknown [12].

It is well known that energy reserves and metabolic conditions play an important role in the timing of pubertal development. Leptin, a hormone released by adipose cells, was first identified in 1994 and is known to play a critical role in body weight homeostasis and the metabolic control of puberty. Patients with mutations in leptin or the leptin receptors have been found to have delayed puberty [13]. The precise mechanism by which leptin influences puberty is not clear, and it may in fact work through an indirect mechanism, possibly through regulation of the KISS1 system [14]. Leptin receptors are highly expressed on kisspeptin neurons. When leptin was administered to leptin-deficient mice, expression of KISS1 increased and puberty was induced [15].

However, this action of leptin on kisspeptin neurons has since been questioned, as LepR knockout mice, in which the leptin receptor was selectively removed from the kisspeptin neurons, still underwent normal puberty [16].

Pubertal Development

Normal pubertal development in girls follows an ordered sequence of events as described by Tanner [17]. Breast development is usually the first sign of puberty. Pubic and axillary hair normally develops about 6 months later, although in a third of girls pubic hair may appear before breast development. Breast development and pubic hair development occur independently, which is a reflection of their underlying driving mechanism. Breast development occurs as a result of rising estradiol levels and pubic and axillary hair by androgen secretion (driven primarily by adrenal glands). Menarche occurs late in puberty, normally corresponding to the end of the growth spurt, when the growth velocity falls below 4cm/year. Maximal growth velocity usually occurs after the start of breast and pubic and axillary hair development, but in some girls the growth spurt may be the first sign of puberty. The complete process of puberty is usually a slow progression, taking a minimum of 18 months [17].

During puberty the ovaries undergo a rapid enlargement as a result of the development of multifollicular cysts under the influence of pulsatile gonadotrophin secretion. The uterus steadily grows through puberty with the body of the uterus gradually becoming longer than the cervix resulting in an adult configuration.

As a result of the relative immaturity of the hypothalamic-pituitary-ovarian axis in the first 2 years following menarche, more than half of menstrual cycles are anovulatory. This results in irregular cycles with cycle frequency varying from less than 20 days to more than 90 days. After the first 1–2 years, the capacity for estrogen-positive feedback on the anterior pituitary develops with the subsequent mid-cycle LH surge and ovulation, resulting in regulation of the menstrual cycle.

Anovulatory cycles are often heavy and prolonged with some girls bleeding for several weeks at a time. This can lead to iron-deficiency anemia, and in rare cases cardiovascular collapse requiring hospital admission and blood transfusion. Initial anovulatory cycles tend to be pain free, although heavy menstrual loss can result in an element of dysmenorrhea. When regular

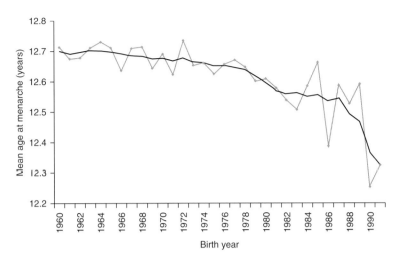

Figure 2.2 Mean age at menarche in 1-year intervals [19].

ovulatory cycles commence, the periods often become more painful because of the increased levels of circulating prostaglandins.

Timing of Puberty

Since the late nineteenth century, the age of onset of puberty has gradually declined, largely the result of improvements in health, nutrition, and sanitation. Onset of puberty is normally based on age at menarche, as this is easy to ascertain. In the UK, the average age of menarche fell from 15 years in 1860 to 13 years in 1960 [18]. A period of stabilization followed until the mid-twentieth century, when another decline began. The 1990–93 cohort in the Breakthrough Generation Study had a mean age of menarche of 12.3 [19]. The onset of puberty can vary by 4–5 years between individuals, with 95 percent of girls showing signs of secondary sexual characteristics between the ages of 8.5 and 13 years (Figure 2.2).

A large US cross-sectional study in 1997 of 17,000 girls in the Pediatric Research in Office Settings network found that 6.7 percent of white girls and 27.2 percent of African American girls had breast or pubic hair development by age 7 [20]. Given this frequency of early breast development, the authors questioned the age criteria for investigating girls for precocious puberty. The study also found that although the average age of breast development was declining, the average age of menarche had stayed relatively stable, resulting in a longer duration of puberty. This study was controversial, however due to concerns of ascertainment bias and lack of thorough breast examination. Current practice in the UK

would be to investigate any girl with signs of pubertal development before age 8.

Childhood obesity is consistently associated with an early onset of puberty. A large prospective cohort study showed that low birth weight and high BMI in childhood were both independently associated with an early age of menarche. When low birth weight and high BMI in childhood were combined, they were associated with the lowest age of menarche in the cohort [21]. The Breakthrough Generations Study looked at factors affecting age of menarche in more than 80,000 women. They found an early age of menarche was associated with low birth weight, maternal preeclampsia, maternal smoking, not being breastfed, nonwhite ethnicity, raised height or weight compared with peers at age 7, and reduced exercise as a child [22]. Endocrine-disrupting chemicals (EDC) are exogenous chemicals that can have an adverse effect on any hormone action. Examples include Bisphenol A (BPA), pesticides, herbicides, and some industrial chemicals. The female reproductive system has been one of the key areas of research over the past 5 years, with some evidence showing an association between EDCs and abnormal puberty. The Endocrine Society has produced two scientific statements on EDCs with recommendations for the future [23].

Variations of Normal

Premature adrenarche is defined as the precocious secretion of adrenal androgens resulting in the appearance of pubic hair (pubarche) before age 8 in girls. Axillary hair, body odor, and acne can occur, but other secondary sexual characteristics are absent. It can be slowly progressive or stay stable, and puberty will usually begin at the normal time. It can be associated with a growth spurt, but the final adult height is unaffected [24]. A retrospective review of 89 children with precocious pubarche showed an association with prematurity, low birth weight, and obesity [25]. Serum androgen concentrations may be slightly raised for chronological age or may be normal. Gonadotrophin levels are prepubertal and bone age is normal.

Premature thelarche is defined as the premature development of breast tissue in the absence of other secondary sexual characteristics before age 8 in girls. The most common age of onset is within the first 2 years of life but can occur at any age. The incidence of progression to precocious puberty has been found to be 14 percent [26]. A more recent study looking at progression in girls presenting with premature thelarche earlier than age 2 found progression in 29 percent [27]. There are various possible mechanisms for premature thelarche, including an increased sensitivity of breast tissue to estrogens, temporary secretion of estrogen from ovarian follicles, increased aromatase activity producing estrogens from androgen precursors, temporary activation of the hypothalamic-pituitary-gonadal axis, and exogenous estrogens. Kisspeptin levels have been found to be raised in girls with premature thelarche, indicating a temporary central activation as a possible cause [28].

Isolated premature menarche is the occurrence of vaginal bleeding in the absence of other secondary sexual characteristics. It is a diagnosis of exclusion after vaginal and uterine pathology, foreign body, and precocious puberty have been ruled out. The mechanisms for isolated premature menarche are the same as for premature thelarche. It can be an isolated event or it can recur. Age of onset of puberty and final adult height are not affected.

When to Investigate

Development of secondary sexual characteristics prior to age 8 should be investigated. Primary amenorrhea is the absence of menarche in a woman otherwise expected to have regular periods and needs to be evaluated in the context of secondary sexual characteristics [29,30,31]. The diagnosis may be made by age 15 if a patient has normal secondary sexual characteristics, or if menarche has failed to occur by 2 years post–breast budding. If secondary sexual characteristics are also absent, diagnosis may be made by age 13 [31].

Psychology and Puberty

As well as the physical changes associated with puberty, there are also significant psychological and emotional changes. Puberty is a time of substantial brain maturation, with gonadal hormones having an effect on many of the neuronal processes [32]. Estrogen has been shown to have an effect on cognitive ability, learning, memory, aggression, and affect regulation [33].

The hypothalamic-pituitary-adrenal (HPA) axis is the primary neuroendocrine axis that mediates the body's response to stress, culminating in the release of cortisol from the adrenal cortex. There are slight alterations in the basal levels of stress hormones during puberty; however, the most dramatic change in the HPA axis occurs following exposure to an acute stressful event. Studies in different animals including humans have shown that females in early adolescence show an increased response of adrenocorticotrophic hormone to stress. This stress reactivity steadily declines in all animals as they progress through puberty into adulthood [34].

Many psychological conditions are associated with adolescence and puberty, including depression, anxiety, eating disorders, antisocial behavior, and risk-taking behavior such as substance misuse [34,35]. Exposure to stressful experiences during pubertal development is thought to play a role in developing these conditions [34].

Conclusion

Embryological and pubertal development in females involves a complex interplay of physiological, genetic, environmental, psychological, and social mechanisms. A sound understanding of this normal process is essential to investigate and manage conditions commonly encountered in pediatric and adolescent gynecology.

References

1. Acien P, Sanchez del Campo F, Mayol M et al. The female gubernaculum: role in the embryology and development of the genital tract and in the possible genesis of malformations. *Eur J Obstet Gynecol Repro Biol.* 2011; **59**: 426–432.

2. Eggers S, Sinclair A. Mammalian sex determination – insights from humans and mice. *Chromosome Res.* 2012; **20**(1): 215–238.

3. Ono M, Harley V. Disorders of sex development: new genes, new concepts. *Nat Rev Endocrinol.* 2013; **9**: 79–91.

4. Arboleda VA, Sandberg DE, Vilain E. DSDs: genetics, underlying pathologies and psychosexual differentiation. *Nat Rev Endocrinol.* 2014; **10**(10): 603–615.

5. Ludbrook LM, Bernard P, Bagheri-Fam S et al. Excess DAX1 leads to XY ovotesticular disorder of sex development (DSD) in mice by inhibiting steroidogenic factor-1 (SF1) activation of the testis enhancer of SRY-box-9 (SOX9). *Endocrinology,* 2012; **153**(4): 1948–1958.

6. Morris DH, Jones ME, Schoemaker MJ et al. Secular trends in age at menarche in women in the UK born 1908–93: results from the breakthrough Generations Study. *Paediatr Perinat Epidemiology.* 2011; **25**(4): 394–400.

7. Kenealy BP, Keen KL, Kapoor A et al. Neuroestradiol in the stalk-median eminence of female rhesus macaques decreases in association with pubertal onset. *Endocrinology.* 2016; **157**: 70–76.

8. DiVall SA, Radovick S. Endocrinology of female puberty. *Curr Opin Endocrinol Diab Obes.* 2009; **16**(1): 1–4.

9. Seminara SB, Messager S, Chatzidaki E et al. The GPR54 Gene as a Regulator of Puberty. *NEJM.* 2003; **349**: 1614–1627.

10. Messager S, Chatzidaki E, Hendrick A et al. Kisspeptin directly stimulates gonadotrophin-receptor hormone release via G protein-coupled receptor. *Proc Natl Acad Sci.* 2005; **54**(102): 1761–1766.

11. Topaloglu AK, Reimann F, Guclu M et al. TAC3 and TACR3 mutations in familial hypogonadotropic hypogonadism reveal a key role for Neurokinin B in the central control of reproduction. *Nat Genet.* 2009; **41**(3): 354–358.

12. Abreu AP, Dauber A, Macedo DB et al. Central precocious puberty caused by mutations in the imprinted gene MKRN3. *N Engl J Med.* 2013; **368**(26): 2467–2475.

13. Strobel A, Issad T, Camoin L et al. A leptin missense mutation associated with hypogonadism and morbid obesity. *Nat Genet.* 1998; **18**: 213–215.

14. Sachez-Garrido MA, Tena-Sempere M. Metabolic control of puberty: roles of leptin and kisspeptins. *Hormones and Behavior.* 2013; **64**(2): 187–194.

15. Smith JT, Acohido BV, Clifton DK et al. KiSS-1 neurones are direct targets for leptin in the ob/ob mouse. *J Neuroendocrinol.* 2006; **18**(4): 298–303.

16. Donato Jr. J, Cravo RM, Frazão R et al. Leptin's effect on puberty in mice is relayed by the ventral premammillary nucleus and does not require signalling in Kiss1 neurons. *J Clin Invest.* 2011; **121**(1): 355–368.

17. Tanner JM. *Foetus into Man: Physical Growth from Conception to Maturity,* 2nd ed. Editor: Tanner JM. Ware: Castlemead, 1989.

18. Marshall WA, Tanner JM. Puberty. In: *Human Growth. A Comprehensive Treatise.* Vol 2. *Postnatal Growth, Neurobiology.* Editors: Falkner F, Tanner JM. London: Plenum Press, 1986; 171–209.

19. Morris DH, Jones ME, Schoemaker MJ et al. Secular trends in age at menarche in women in the UK born 1908–93: results from the breakthrough Generations Study. *Paediatr Perinat Epidemiology.* 2011; **25**(4): 394–400.

20. Herman-Giddens M, Slora E, Wasserman R et al. Secondary sexual characteristics and menses in young girls seen in office practice: a study from the pediatric research in office settings network. *Pediatrics* 1997; **99**: 505–512.

21. Sloboda DM, Hart R, Doherty DA et al. Age at menarche: influences of prenatal and postnatal growth. *J Clin Endocrinol Metab* 2007; **92**: 46–50.

22. Morris DH, Jones ME, Schoemaker MJ et al. Determinants of age at menarche in the UK: analyses from the breakthrough Generations Study. *Br J Cancer.* 2010; **103**(11): 1760–1764.

23. Gore AC, Chappell VA, Fenton SE et al. EDC-2: The Endocrine Society's Second Scientific Statement on Endocrine-Disrupting Chemicals. *Endocr Rev.* 2015; **36**(6): E1–E150.

24. Leung A, Robson LM. Premature adrenarche. *J Paed Health Care.* 2008; **22**(4): 230–233.

25. Neville KA, Walker JL. Precocious pubarche is associated with SGA, prematurity, weight gain and obesity. *Arch Dis Child.* 2005; **90**: 258–261.

26. Pasquino AM, Pucarelli I, Passeri F et al. Progression of premature thelarche to central precocious puberty. *J Pediatr.* 1995; **126**(1): 11–14.

27. Ucar A, Saka N, Bas F et al. Is premature thelarche in the first two years of life transient? *J Clin Res Pediatr Endocrinol.* 2012; **4**(3): 140–145.

28. Akinci A, Cetin D, Ilhan N. Plasma kisspeptin levels in girls with premature thelarche. *J Clin Res Pediatr Endocrinol.* 2012; **4**(2): 61–65.

29. Marshall WA, Tanner JM. Variations in pattern of pubertal changes in girls. *Arch Dis Child.* 1969; **44**(235): 291–303.

30. Warren MP, Hagey AR. The genetics, diagnosis and treatment of amenorrhea. *Minerva Ginecol.* 2004; **56**(5): 437–455.

31. American Society for Reproductive Medicine, Practice Committee. Current evaluation of amenorrhea. *Fertil Steril.* 2008; **90**(5 Suppl): S219–25.

32. McEwen BS, Alves SE. Estrogen actions in the central nervous system. *Endocrine Rev.* 2003; **20**: 279–307.

33. Cameron JL. Interrelationships between hormones, behavior, and affect during adolescence. *Ann N Y Acad Sci.* 2004; **1021**: 110–123.

34. Romeo RD. Pubertal maturation and programming of hypothalamic-pituitary-adrenal reactivity. *Front Neuroendocrinol.* 2010; **31**(2): 232–240.

35. Patton GC, Viner R. Pubertal transitions in health. *Lancet.* 2007; **369**: 1130–1139.

Holistic Assessment in Pediatric and Adolescent Gynecology Practice
Gynecological History Taking and Clinical Examination in the Child and Adolescent

Paul L. Wood and Jennie Yoost

The History

A pediatric and adolescent gynecology (PAG) clinical history and examination require both the expertise of a pediatrician in terms of communicating and engaging with a child and the expertise of a gynecologist in addressing sensitive and intimate issues that inevitably form part of such an assessment. The first pelvic examination experienced by an adolescent may shape her future approach to reproductive health issues.

The child must remain at the center of the interaction and her interests must always come first, although the parent or guardian often leads in the interaction. The circumstances under which a history is taken for the first time therefore requires an appropriate environment. Children with gynecological problems should not be seen in the setting of an adult gynecology clinic. There should instead be a designated regular PAG clinic supported by a pediatric and/or specialist nurse [1], the presence of whom is important in terms of support, often providing a different perspective to the consultation from that of the gynecologist.

With young children it may be best for the pediatric nurse to usher the child into the consultation room with the parent or care provider before meeting the gynecologist so that the child can be introduced to the surroundings and begin playing. Distraction tools are important in a PAG consultation. Once the child has settled, then the gynecologist can introduce himself/herself, greeting the child and asking the child to introduce her parent or care provider. Questions need to be posed according to the child's age, understanding, and development, but simple questions can be addressed to the child alternating with the adult who can provide answers to other more complex questions. In this way the child is absorbed into the consultation. The younger the child the more reliable the answers can be. In addition, parental anxiety can impair communication in the course of the consultation. An empathetic approach by the gynecologist is more likely to improve communication.

The structure employed when taking a child's medical history may differ from that with an adult. With adults the history of the presenting complaint is often addressed first. With children it may prove helpful to start by asking general questions such as past medical and family history to set the scene and help relax and engage the child before addressing the often more sensitive reasons for the visit.

The history should include pregnancy and birth details, developmental milestones, family history, and safeguarding issues. The clinician should remain open minded throughout and not necessarily accept all the information given at face value – for instance, what is purported to have been the menarche might not have been the first menstrual period at all. Child protection needs to be at the forefront of all PAG consultations. All the information provided needs to be absorbed and fully documented for future reference.

Language used must be age and developmentally appropriate. Children use proper names for other body parts, and there should not be any particular part of the body that is designated as being too shameful to call by its proper name. Whereas best practice should be to encourage accurate anatomical descriptors, the clinician should nevertheless be aware of alternative terms familiar to that particular child. In one retrospective study exploring children's knowledge of human genital anatomy, only 6.1 percent of females learned correct names for female genitalia. Female respondents did not complete their anatomical vocabulary for female genitalia until a mean age of 15.6 years [2]. Clinical terminology should also accord with the Chicago Consensus 2011 [3]. The use of new terms under the umbrella of disorders of sex development was believed to improve communication and parental understanding while being acceptable to affected individuals [4]. This approach appears to have been accepted by participants including parents with broad support for the terminology.

Different approaches are needed when interacting with adolescents. The gynecologist should try and avoid being paternalistic and didactic, yet maintain a comfortable patient-clinician relationship. Introductions can be on first name terms, difficult as it might be to those clinicians used to more formal introductions. Questions should be open ended so that "yes/no" answers can be avoided and the adolescent encouraged to express herself. The gynecologist should follow the one-minute rule when speaking to an adolescent and limit the time spent talking at any one time to no more than a minute.

The HEADSS [5] framework (Home, Education, Activity, Drugs, Sexuality, Suicide/Depression) first introduced in 1972, is a useful tool to aid consultations with adolescents and provides an opportunity to facilitate rapport and risk assessment (Table 3A.1). A psychosocial review of systems is considered to be essential and to be at least as important as the physical examination. The framework develops from expected and less threatening questions to more personal and intrusive questions, allowing the clinician an opportunity to establish trust and rapport with the adolescent before addressing more difficult questions. In particular, difficult questions should be best presented in a factual and nonjudgmental manner (e.g., while exploring any current relationship, also ask "when was the last time you had sex with anyone else?").

Adolescents often attend the consultation with a parent or guardian, and this can influence the extent to which sensitive matters can be broached. The gynecologist should try and engage with the parent but focus on the presenting complaint and accompanying story. The sexual history is crucial, with many parents volunteering (often mistakenly) that mother and daughter are completely open in such matters. Using the line that the adolescent probably has friends who are sexually active is a potential icebreaker, allowing for anonymity in front of the parent. In this respect there is no harm in inquiring about the sexual history with the mother present, but the clinician should engineer an opportunity to speak to the adolescent

Table 3A.1 HEADSS mnemonic (adapted)

H	Home	Living arrangements
		Transience
		Relationships with carers/ significant others
		Community support
		Supervision
		Abuse
		Childhood experiences
		Cultural identity
		Recent life events
E	Education	School/work retention and relationships
	Employment	Bullying
	Eating	Study/career progression and goals
	Exercise	Nutrition
		Eating patterns
		Weight change
		Exercise, fitness, and energy
A	Activities	Hobbies
	Hobbies	Peer activities and venues
	Peer relationships	Lifestyle factors
		Risk taking
		Injury avoidance
D	Drug use	Alcohol
		Tobacco
		Caffeine
		Prescription
		Recreational
S	Sexual activity	Sexual activity
	Sexuality	Age onset
	Safety from injury, exploitation, trafficking, grooming, and violence	Safe-sex practices
		Same-sex attraction
		STI screening
		Sexual abuse
		Pregnancy
S	Suicide	Depression
	Depression	Anxiety
	Mental health	Reactions to stress
		Risk assessment
		Suicidal ideation/intent

alone to allow her to share her history with the assurance of patient confidentiality.

Discussing confidentiality at the forefront of the visit can be helpful in managing expectations of the parent and patient. A model visit with an adolescent patient can include a time of discussion with both parent and patient together, followed by a confidential discussion with the patient alone.

If a new disclosure relating to sexual abuse is made during the course of the consultation, more detailed questioning should cease and immediate contact made with the local child protection/safeguarding team to enable the child's immediate safety and arrange for a formal interview to take place. It is only once the clinician has satisfied himself/herself with the history that an examination of the child or adolescent is offered.

The Examination

Young females may be anxious about a pelvic examination, for fear of discomfort, or embarrassment about the nature of the exam. For this reason, it is imperative that the clinician is candid about the examination, explains what is proposed, and approaches it in a calm and unrushed manner. A gynecologic examination is an excellent opportunity to provide education to the patient and parents about anatomy, hygiene, physiology, and safe and healthy practices. An explanation upfront about what will be done, before the patient undresses, can place the patient at ease. This explanation should include a stepwise account of the examination and what tools will be used (stirrups, cotton swabs, directed lighting, specula). Younger children may want to visualize and handle these tools as well. For many gynecologic concerns, especially at a younger age, instrumentation of the vagina is not necessary, and addressing this beforehand can be reassuring to the patient and parent.

Before the examination begins, the clinician should assess who should be present. In younger children, typically one parent stays with the child, but the child may want both parents or other family present. Older adolescents may feel more comfortable with family waiting outside during the examination allowing for an opportunity to broach confidential matters. This decision should be at the discretion of the patient. It is also important to assess the cooperativeness of the patient. For a non-urgent problem, an examination can be deferred, and the patient can be brought back for another visit when she is more prepared for an examination. In some cases, several visits may occur before an examination is performed, which allows building of trust and clinician rapport.

The Pediatric Exam

Although many children will have undergone physical clinical examinations previously, a detailed gynecological examination presents different challenges and a new experience for the child. A younger child can be positioned in a variety of ways to facilitate

(a)

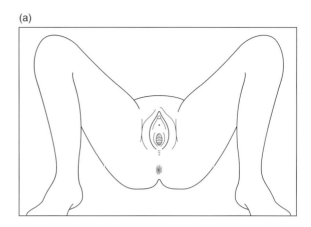

(b)

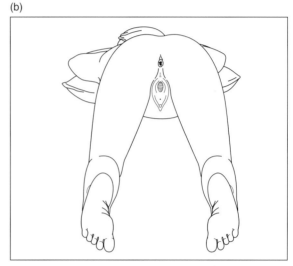

Figure 3A.1 Positioning of a pediatric patient

a gynecologic exam (Figure 3A.1). The comfort of the child during the positioning should always be assessed. Stirrups may be used, but it is probably best for the child to be asked to place her legs "like a frog" or "like a butterfly" with the heels of her feet together. The knee-chest position can also be used. Good lighting is essential. The parent or guardian should be involved in this process and can even sit with the child on the exam table or have the child in his or her lap in the frog-leg position. The child can also assist in the exam by helping spread the labia or pointing to the area of concern.

All external structures should be evaluated and documented in detail avoiding subjective comment (e.g., intact hymen), instead providing an accurate anatomical description. Visual inspection includes assessment of the skin, labia majora, labia minora, clitoris and clitoral hood, urethra, hymen, perineum,

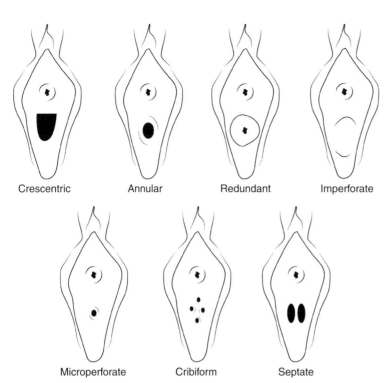

Figure 3A.2 Variations in hymen anatomy

and anus. This also includes Tanner staging of pubertal development. The skin of the vulva should be assessed for signs of lesions, excoriation, hygiene issues, or inflammation. The hymen can be better visualized with gentle downward and outward traction on the labia majora. This motion also allows assessment of the lower vagina, which can assist in evaluation of discharge, trauma, or foreign body. The hymen in prepubertal females should be unestrogenized and is normally annular, crescentric, or redundant [6].

Proper visualization is important to rule out anomalies such as septate, microperforate, cribiform, or imperforate hymens (Figure 3A.2). Documentation should be descriptive to facilitate future exams and determine whether change is present. The use of a diagram for documentation can be useful (Figure 3A.3).

Collection of vaginal samples can be done a variety of ways. It is important to remember that the hymenal tissue is very sensitive, and a cotton tip applicator can cause significant discomfort in young females. For vaginal collections, the use of a small-caliber urethral swab should be used with labial traction to access the vagina and avoid contact with the hymen. Topical lidocaine ointment can be placed at the introitus prior to collection of samples. Alternatively, the vagina can

be irrigated with saline using a nasogastric tube or a butterfly catheter with needle removed, placed within a pediatric red rubber catheter [7]. This can be helpful in retrieving foreign bodies. Cotton swabs can be placed at the introitus to collect irrigated fluid. This is rarely required.

Rectal examination should really be avoided altogether unless considered to be absolutely necessary. The use of noninvasive imaging such as ultrasound should replace the need for a rectal examination.

At the conclusion of the examination, the child should be thanked and praised for her cooperation. Education regarding anatomy, pubertal development, hygiene, and findings on examination can then be discussed in detail with the guardian and child. The use of pictures can assist in the description of the exam and therapy, especially if medication application or monitoring is needed with parental involvement.

Adolescent Exam

In adolescents, a pelvic examination can sometimes be a barrier for seeking care. Adolescents may see a gynecologist for many reasons that do not require a pelvic examination including contraception initiation. Sexual

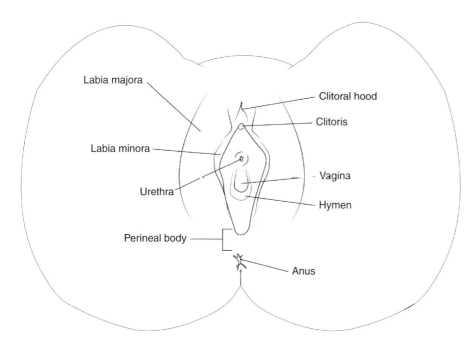

Figure 3A.3 Anatomy diagram for documentation or for patient education

activity does not mandate a pelvic exam, and a pelvic exam is not likely to detect conditions for which a patient would not be a candidate for hormonal contraception. Hormonal contraception can be safely provided based on a thorough medical history and blood pressure measurement [8]. However, a gynecologic exam for adolescents is an optimal time to discuss normal anatomy and preventative care. Many adolescents may have questions about their appearance or sexual function that they may be embarrassed to ask. Providing education and reassuring them about their anatomy during an exam will put the patient at ease and facilitate future conversation.

The examination should begin with an assessment of the body mass index (and plotting of height and weight on centile charts), blood pressure measurement as necessary, abdominal palpation, and inspection of external vulval structures. This includes Tanner staging and assessment of skin thereby promoting discussion about shaving safety, presence of folliculitis, vulvar hygiene, and normal leukorrhea. Assessment of normal sebaceous glands, nevi, and papillomatosis can also be reviewed with the patient. Hymen anatomy in adolescents shows signs of estrogenization, and the hymen appears plump and pale pink compared to a redder and more delicate hymen in prepubertal females.

Labia minora change in size and thickness with puberty and may become asymmetric. Studies evaluating labial size show that labial width can range from 3 to 50 mm in the adult population [9]. Adolescents may be concerned about the size or shape of their labia due to lack of variation among media images, or increased prevalence of labiaplasty. Measurement of the labia with a tape measure can help to provide an objective assessment for the adolescent. Education and reassurance are key to managing these concerns, along with discussion of conservative measures to reduce irritation. This includes fragrance-free soaps, use of bland emollients, cotton underwear, and cessation of vulvar shaving [9].

Swabs for vaginitis can be obtained without a speculum and testing for sexually transmitted infections can be performed with vaginal swabs or on urine samples using nucleic acid amplification tests (NAATs). In sexually active adolescents, yearly screening for gonorrhea and chlamydia is recommended in the United States until age 25, and with any new risk factor such as a new sexual partner [10]. The use of NAATs has high sensitivity and specificity for both gonorrhea and chlamydia on both urine specimens and endocervical samples [11].

The performance of a speculum exam and bimanual examination should again be dictated by the chief complaint. In adolescents, a smaller speculum such as a Huffman or Pederson is typically used. Collection of a Pap smear is not indicated until after adolescence regardless of sexual debut [12], and the discussion of what this testing is and when it should be obtained should occur. Bimanual examination can be performed using a single digit or two digits to palpate the adnexa and uterus. Other structures can also be palpated including the urethra, bladder, and muscles of the pelvic floor. A rectovaginal exam can also be used to assess higher in the pelvis posterior to the uterus. At the conclusion of the exam, all findings should be discussed with the patient, with reassurance and explanation of any abnormal findings.

In summary, a holistic approach is required for the taking of a history and the performance of a gynecological examination in children and adolescents. Appropriate measures are needed to ensure that as much relevant information is obtained that will aid with the management of the presenting gynecological complaint.

References

1. BritSPAG. Clinical Standards for Service Planning in PAG. January 2011. Britspag.org

2. Gartrell N, Mosbacher D Sex differences in the naming of children's genitalia. *Sex Roles*. 1984; **10**(11): 869–76.

3. Hughes IA, Houk C, Ahmed SF et al. LWPES Consensus Group; ESPE Consensus Group. Consensus statement on management of intersex disorders. *Arch Dis Child*. 2006; **91**: 554–63.

4. Davies JG, Knight EJ, Savage A et al. Evaluation of terminology used to describe disorders of sex development. *J Pediatr Urol* 2011; **7**(4): 412–415.

5. Goldenring JM, Rosen DS. Getting into adolescent heads: an essential update. *Contemp Pediatr*. 2004; **21**(1): 64–90.

6. Heger AH, Ticson L, Lister J et al . Appearance of the genitalia in girls selected for nonabuse: review of hymenal morphology and nonspecific findings. *J Pediatr Adolesc Gynecol*. 2002; **15**(1): 27–35.

7. Rome ES Vulvovaginitis and other common vulvar disorders in children. *Endocr Dev*. 2012; **22**: 72–83.

8. Stewart FH, Harper CC, Ellertson CE et al. Clinical breast and pelvic examination requirements for hormonal contraception: Current practice vs evidence. *JAMA*. 2001; **285**(17): 2232–39.

9. Runacres SA, Wood PL. Cosmetic labiaplasty in an adolescent population. *J Pediatr Adolesc Gynecol*. 2015. DOI: 10.1016/j.jpag.2015.09.010.

10. Centers for Disease Control and Prevention. Recommendations for the laboratory-based detection of Chlamydia trachomatis and Neisseria gonorrhoeae – 2014. *MMWR Recomm Rep*. 2014; **63**(RR-02): 1–19.

11. LeFevre ML. Screening for chlamydia and gonorrhoea: US Preventive Services Task Force Recommendation Statement. *Annals of Internal Medicine*. 2014; **161**(12): 902–10.

12. American College of Obstetricians and Gynecologists. Practice Bulletin No. 140: Management of abnormal cervical cancer screening test results and cervical cancer precursors. *Obstet Gynecol*. 2013; **122**(6): 1338–67.

Holistic Assessment in Pediatric and Adolescent Gynecology Practice
Imaging in Pediatric and Adolescent Gynecology

Margaret Hall-Craggs and Davor Jurkovic

Introduction

Imaging is used to supplement the clinical and biochemical assessment of children and adolescents presenting with gynecological abnormalities. A key concern is to avoid the use of ionizing radiation in these young patients and consequently ultrasound (US) and magnetic resonance imaging (MRI) are the most commonly used imaging modalities. Ultrasound is used in the vast majority of cases as first-line imaging assessment supplemented by MRI when necessary.

Principles of Ultrasound and MRI

What Is Ultrasound?

Ultrasound (US) is a diagnostic technique that uses sound waves at high frequency to generate images of internal organs. In the pediatric gynecological patient, US examination is performed transabdominally (TAS), using a full bladder as the ultrasonic window. Good views cannot always be achieved if the bladder is under-filled, overlying bowel gas is present, extensive pelvic adhesions fix loops of bowel to pelvic organs, or complex bladder and bowel anomalies are present.

TAS is usually performed using a curvilinear probe with varying frequencies depending on the age of the patient; 7.5 MHz transducers are used in neonates and 5 MHz transducers in children and adolescents, facilitating better views of deeply pelvic organs. In sexually active adolescents, transvaginal ultrasound (TVS) is the preferred route.

Transperineal ultrasound (TPS) is useful where there is a transverse vaginal septum. Transrectal scans (TRS) should be considered in virgin adolescents when determining the nature of the pelvic abnormality is critical for further management, and diagnosis cannot be made using other diagnostic modalities [1].

Ultrasound is a widely available, simple, and inexpensive diagnostic modality, which makes it ideal for the initial assessment of both pediatric and adult gynecological patients. It is operator dependent and the diagnostic performance is determined by locally available expertise. In optimal circumstances ultrasound provides sufficient information to solve most routine diagnostic problems in pediatric gynecology.

What Is MRI?

Magnetic resonance imaging is a method of creating images by placing the patient in a strong magnetic field, commonly around 1.5 Tesla, and pulsing the body with radiofrequency (RF) waves. The body is transparent to RF waves, so they can pass through the body tissue and interact with it. MRI images protons (hydrogen atoms) and in the human body the vast majority of these are in water, with a smaller number in fat. The absorption of energy from the RF waves is determined by the nature of the molecules that the protons are bound to and their environment. The energy is re-emitted by the body and the pattern reflects the type of tissue the protons are in, and their position in space. Consequently a picture of the body can be built up in two or sometimes three-dimensional slices, reflecting water and fat distribution and their environment within the body tissue.

MRI uses non-ionizing low-energy radiation and therefore is safer than CT scans (which use higher energy X-rays), when used in a controlled fashion. Some people cannot have an MR scan. For example, some brain implants and cardiac pacing wires are not suitable for MR scanning and can move, be damaged, or generate local heat.

Babies, children, and adolescents can be assessed with MRI. Most can be scanned with just some preliminary preparation from radiographers and play specialists. A few patients cannot tolerate the noise or being inside the scanner; they may need sedation or general anesthesia. Babies can be fed, wrapped, and mildly sedated, if indicated, for scans.

An advantage of MRI is that the images are generally easier for clinicians to interpret compared to ultrasound. Repeat scans can produce equivalent images facilitating easier follow-up.

The key to high-quality MRI studies is multiplanar imaging with appropriate scan planes, sequences, high-resolution images of the pelvis, and generally the use of gadolinium contrast agent. Images are vastly improved by the use of buscopan/glucagon to suppress bowel motion artifact, and propellor sequences that reduce movement artifacts.

By the time patients are imaged with MRI, there is usually a provisional diagnosis made clinically and by diagnostic ultrasound; MRI is generally used to provide confirmatory and supplementary information. For example, it might be used to confirm and stage tumors, to confirm a diagnosis of ovarian torsion, and to fully describe the abnormalities of urogynecological congenital anomalies.

Normal Pelvic Anatomy

The uterus and ovaries undergo changes in size and morphology during childhood and adolescence affecting their appearance.

The Uterus

During the neonatal period, the uterus is enlarged and the endometrium appears as a clear echogenic stripe because of the influence of in-utero stimulation by maternal hormones. In 25 percent of neonates, a small amount of fluid is present within the endometrial cavity. The uterus is usually "spade-shaped," measures approximately 3.5 cm in length and the cervix is larger than the fundus (ratio 2:1). As circulating maternal hormones decline, after three months the uterus regresses to around 2.5–3 cm in length with equal corpus-cervix ratio, and it can be tubular.

The uterus gradually increases in length to 4.5 cm between ages 2 and 8. From puberty onward, the uterus develops the adult pear shape and measures 5–8 cm. The corpus-cervix ratio approaches 3:1 and the endometrium demonstrates fluctuations in thickness and echogenicity in response to the menstrual cycle. Color Doppler usually detects blood flow within the myometrium but little or no flow in the endometrium [2].

On MRI, the postpubertal adolescent uterus shows a three-layered corpus and a one- or two-layered cervical stroma. There is a T2 high-signal center that represents the endometrial stripe. Surrounding this is the junctional zone, and superficial to this is the myometrium. The cervical stroma can consist of a single low-signal layer, with a very small high-signal center due to the endocervix. However, the stroma can also consist of a low-signal ring around the endocervical canal with an intermediate signal layer superficial to it, very similar to and blending with the myometrial layer of the corpus.

The Ovary

The normal neonatal ovarian volume is usually around 1 ml, becoming smaller in the second year of life resulting from declining maternal hormones. Ovaries can be located anywhere along their embryological course from the lower pole of the kidney to the broad ligament. Follicles can be visualized in up to 84 percent of cases from birth to 24 months in age and in 68 percent of cases between ages 2 and 12 [3]. The ovaries remain quiescent until the age 6. Thereafter, the ovarian volume in premenarchal girls increases to 1.2–4 ml.

In postmenarchal girls ovarian volume increases to an average of 8–9 ml and typically contains a large number of antral and maturing follicles in each menstrual cycle. In addition, the ovary develops into an ovoid shape in response to circulating gonadotropins and appears located deeper into the pelvis.

The Vagina

The vagina is well seen on both ultrasound and MRI. Ultrasound is useful for the diagnosis of foreign bodies and when there is no obvious vaginal introitus. The length of the vagina can be assessed on MRI by measuring the distance between the most proximal portion of the vagina and its distal margin, which is marked by the urethral meatus [4]. The vagina is best seen on transverse images using either small field of view (FOV) transverse T2 weighted scans or post-contrast T1 images. An assessment of the size of the clitoris can be made, but this is not really essential as it is usually inspected clinically.

The Role of Imaging in Specific Clinical Problems

Prepubertal Bleeding

Ultrasound is an effective way of screening for various causes of prepubertal vaginal bleeding such as foreign bodies or tumor. In central precocious puberty, the uterine and ovarian volumes are increased due to the effect of increased gonadotropins. In these cases MRI or CT of the brain should be considered to detect intracranial causes of disease. Posttreatment ultrasound can be used for follow-up to demonstrate that the uterus and ovaries have returned to normal.

The most common cause of peripheral precocious puberty (PPP) is autonomous follicular cysts often seen on ultrasound as a unilateral follicular ovarian cyst with a "daughter cyst sign" representing an adjacent antral follicle. The stimulated uterus has a pubertal appearance. Estrogen-secreting tumors causing PPP are discussed later.

Primary Amenorrhea

The imaging investigation of primary amenorrhea follows exclusion of nonstructural causes, such as hormonal dysfunction and anorexia. The imaging pathway is determined by the presence or absence of secondary sexual characteristics and/or pain. Initial ultrasound can show whether there is an underlying anatomical cause for amenorrhea and can also be used to evaluate the renal system to identify coexisting anomalies. MRI of primary amenorrhea is used where diagnostic ultrasound is not definitive.

Painless Primary Amenorrhea

The most common cause for primary painless amenorrhea is gonadal dysgenesis. TAS will often show a normal prepubertal uterus and ovaries vary from non-visualized streak ovaries to a normal appearance. The investigation of patients for whom congenital anomalies are the cause of the primary amenorrhea is discussed later. The most common MRI diagnosed causes of primary amenorrhea are complete androgen insensitivity syndrome (CAIS) and Mayer-Rokitansky-Kuster-Hauser (MRKH) syndrome.

Painful Primary Amenorrhea

Most cases are secondary to obstructed menstruation, which can be due to an imperforate hymen or

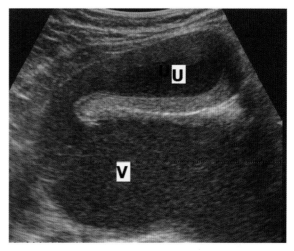

Figure 3B.1 A transabdominal ultrasound scan on a 15-year-old girl presenting with primary amenorrhea and intermittent lower abdominal pain. On longitudinal view the vagina (V) and the uterus (U) are distended with a large amount of blood. The diagnosis of imperforate hymen was confirmed on clinical examination and at surgery.

transverse vaginal septum. Ultrasound and MRI can show the level of obstruction and detect concomitant Mullerian anomalies. Real-time ultrasound can be used to guide incision of vaginal septum or cervical dilatation (Figure 3B.1).

Pelvic Pain

There are a multitude of causes of pelvic pain, and these will largely be assessed by a combination of clinical examination and ultrasound. Pain in the pediatric/adolescent female may be cyclical, non-cyclical, or acute. Gynecological causes of pelvic pain include ovarian torsion and obstructed menstruation. The latter case can be associated with primary amenorrhea, such as a transverse vaginal septum, or with menstruation, such as in patients with an obstructed hemivagina, or functioning non-communicating unicornuate uterus (Figure 3B.2).

Ultrasound is used as the primary imaging tool for assessing pelvic pain but MRI can sometimes help diagnose other causes such as infection, appendicitis, mesenteric adenitis, and inflammatory bowel disease.

Ovarian Torsion

Torsion can occur if there are predisposing factors such as ovarian cysts or masses, but also in the normal ovary due to excess mobility and a relatively long

23

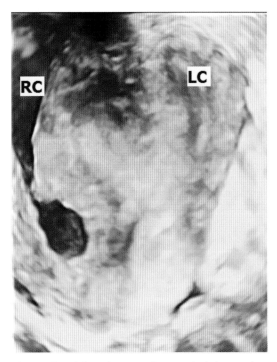

Figure 3B.2 A three-dimensional transvaginal ultrasound scan in a 19-year-old woman presenting with severe dysmenorrhea. The diagnosis of bicornuate uterus was made. The left uterine cornu (LC) is well developed and contains thin endometrium. The right cornu (RC) is also well formed but it is distended with blood due to an obstructed hemivagina.

Fallopian tube. The US and MR features of torsion can be variable and should be combined with clinical assessment. Signs include the following:

- Unilateral enlargement of the ovary with associated stromal edema (Figure 3B.3)
- Ill-defined borders
- Peripheral arrangement of the follicles, more prominent in prepubertal girls [4]
- A twisted ovarian pedicle

In some cases, US-guided aspiration of a simple cyst torsion can be used as an immediate and interim measure for management [5].

Hemorrhagic Cysts and Rupture

In menstruating girls, acute cyclical mid-cycle pelvic pain is often related to follicular and functional hemorrhagic ovarian cysts. The hemorrhagic content can show a debris-fluid level and coagulated blood clots. Occasionally there may also be evidence of free fluid or hemoperitoneum, seen as echogenic thick fluid in the pelvis on ultrasound or high signal on T1-weighted MR images. These cysts usually

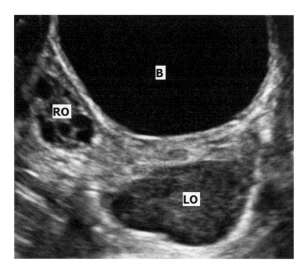

Figure 3B.3 Ultrasound transverse view of a pelvis in an 8-year-old girl presenting with acute left iliac fossa pain. The right ovary (RO) appears normal while the left ovary (LO) is enlarged with a marked stromal edema. These findings are typical of ovarian torsion.

resolve spontaneously and can be managed expectantly, unless there is hemodynamic instability.

Partial Obstruction to Menstrual Flow

Partial obstruction can also be a cause of cyclical pelvic pain in duplex systems, where blood collects in the obstructed hemivagina but menstruation is preserved due to a functioning non-obstructed side.

Imaging of Pelvic Tumors

Gynecological causes of pelvic masses in children and adolescents include tumors and obstructed menstruation. Obstructed menstruation with distension of the gynecological tract due to tubo-ovarian masses or distended uterus or vagina can present as a painful mass with or without primary amenorrhea.

Benign pelvic tumors are most commonly assessed with ultrasound, and MRI is usually reserved for cases where there is diagnostic uncertainty. In malignant pelvic tumors affecting children and adolescents, MRI can show the primary tumor and evidence of spread, particularly to other pelvic organs and lymph nodes (Figure 3B.4). Omental disease and ascites may be apparent, but peritoneal disease is difficult to see unless it is fairly extensive.

Benign Ovarian Cysts and Tumors

The majority of ovarian cysts in children and adolescents are benign and may present with pain. Large

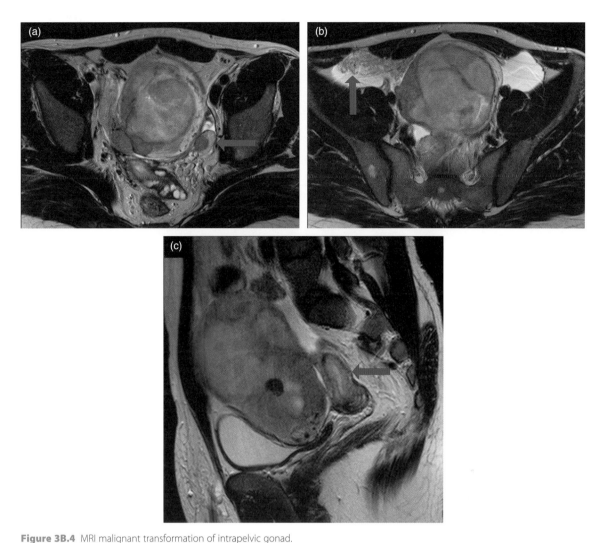

Figure 3B.4 MRI malignant transformation of intrapelvic gonad.
Transverse T2-weighted (a and b) and sagittal T2 weighted MRI (c) scans of the pelvis.
The right intrapelvic testis in this patient with a DSD has undergone malignant change and is seen as a large mass in the center of the pelvis. The left intrapelvic testis (arrowed, a) contains a low-signal eccentric Sertoli adenoma. There is pelvic ascites and an omental cake (arrowed, b). In addition to testes, this phenotypically male patient had a small midline uterus (arrowed, c).

ovarian cysts usually peak at two periods: in the first year of life and around menarche. After puberty, benign cysts are usually either follicular or functional cysts measuring up to 10 cm. These can resolve spontaneously. Corpus luteum cysts can also be painful and hemorrhagic.

Dermoid cysts are the most common type of benign ovarian tumors, accounting for up to 75 percent of cases. These present between ages 6 and 15, and 10 percent are bilateral; many are found as incidental findings. These cysts are often of mixed echogenicity on ultrasound with acoustic shadowing, due to calcifications or a mixture of sebum, hair, and teeth.

On MRI they show mixed fat, water, and low-signal nodules shaped as teeth (Figure 3B.5).

Malignant Tumors

Ovarian neoplasms are uncommon in children and adolescents. Although ultrasound by an experienced operator can raise the suspicion of a malignancy as well as yielding a conclusive diagnosis, additional imaging with MRI is often required to assess metastatic disease.

Granulosa cell tumors (GCT) are the most common form of sex cord stromal tumors. Juvenile GCTs have a different appearance when compared to adult

25

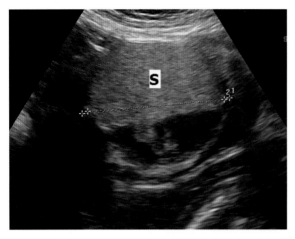

Figure 3B.5 A transabdominal ultrasound scan showing a large dermoid cyst with a well-defined fluid level. The fluid in the upper part of the cyst is bright and echogenic, which is typical of sebum (S).

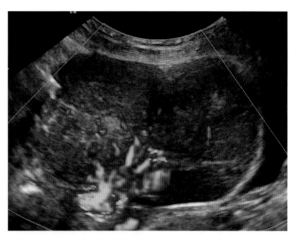

Figure 3B.6 A large unilateral solid pelvic tumor that appeared highly vascular on ultrasound Doppler examination. These findings were typical of a non-epithelial malignant ovarian tumor. The diagnosis of dysgerminoma was confirmed on histology.

GCT and are seen as mainly solid complex masses. They are typically highly vascular on Doppler sonography and contrast enhancement on MRI.

Immature teratomas are the most common type of malignant germ cell tumors and can be bilateral in 12 percent to 15 percent of cases. They are heterogeneous, predominantly solid masses, which may have cystic spaces filled with mucinous or serous fluid. Dysgerminomas tend to be solid tumors with a lobulated structure, an irregular internal echogenicity, but well-defined external borders. They are also highly vascular on Doppler examination. Other types of non-epithelial ovarian tumors are rare in childhood and tend to also be mainly solid and highly vascular masses (Figure 3B.6).

Sarcomas, such as rhabdomyosarcoma of the vagina, are rare tumors that may occur in the young and are commonly imaged using both ultrasound and MRI for assessment of the primary tumor and disease staging. Occasionally malignant disease is seen in the pelvis due to metastatic tumor from other primaries.

Pregnancy and Pelvic Inflammatory Disease

In sexually active teenagers, it is important to consider pregnancy and pelvic inflammatory disease as causes for pelvic pain. TVS can diagnose early pregnancy and exclude ectopic pregnancy. In pelvic inflammatory disease, imaging can show a pyosalpinx or tubo-ovarian abscess.

Imaging of Congenital Anomalies

Ultrasound is invariably used as first line of imaging in most patients presenting with primary amenorrhea, pelvic pain, a mass, or suspected anomaly. It is often sufficient to detect congenital uterine anomalies particularly with the advent of transvaginal three-dimensional ultrasound.

However, for complex anomalies MRI is extremely useful and it can also assess associated skeletal, renal, urological, and neural abnormalities at the same time. Multiplanar or three-dimensional imaging allows complex anatomy to be unraveled. The sequences used can be tailored to show altered blood, and gadolinium contrast agents can help show highly vascularized tissue such as the vagina.

The main purposes of imaging in congenital anomalies are as follows:

1. To diagnose the abnormality and to classify it
2. To define anatomy
3. To identify primary or postoperative complications including obstruction
4. To aid pre-surgical planning
5. To assess associated abnormalities
6. To help assess the potential for fertility

Some anomalies are very complex but high-quality imaging can define the anatomy. In addition to helping plan surgery, MRI scans can contribute to assessing the potential for fertility, such as defining the presence and adequacy of the cervix, and the presence of functioning endometrium. Careful assessment for other associated anomalies such as renal anomalies and the presence of ureteric remnants is helpful for surgical planning [6]. Measurement of the vagina and the length of any vaginal defects is helpful for defining the nature and approach of reconstructive surgery.

In complicated uterine anomalies, such as duplex system where there is a double uterus and an obstructed hemivagina, intraoperative ultrasound can be helpful in guiding drainage and subsequent dilatation of the vagina

Specific Congenital Anomalies

Unicornuate Uterus

The appearance of a unicornuate uterine anomaly can vary from a single lateralized functioning uterine horn with visualization of the ipsilateral ovary only, to more complex cases where there may be a communicating or noncommunicating horn, which may or may not be functional. In many cases, the diagnosis can be made by two-dimensional ultrasound scan. The presence of blood can also be seen in a functional rudimentary horn, and this may be a cause of cyclical pelvic pain.

In complex cases of unicornuate uterus, where there may be a functioning noncommunicating

rudimentary horn, MRI can show the presence of blood distending the rudimentary cornu. It can also show the site and extent of the attachment of the rudimentary horn to the dominant unicornuate horn. This is extremely helpful for pre-surgical planning as the more extensive the attachment, the more difficult the surgery. In addition, demonstration of the relationship of the rudimentary horn to the cervix of the dominate horn is helpful to the surgeon in planning conservation of the cervix, protecting the integrity of the residual uterus in terms of its potential for fertility.

Septate Uterus

Ultrasound and MRI of the septate uterus can show the extent of the septum (partial or complete). MRI can also demonstrate the composition of the septum, which can be muscular proximally, merging with the fundal myometrium, and fibrous distally. Definition of the muscular/fibrous boundary is helpful for pre-surgical planning as resection is limited to the fibrous portion of the septum (Figure 3B.7). For those who require surgery, intraoperative ultrasound is useful to increase the efficacy and safety of resection. Postoperative scans provide an effective way of determining the success of surgery and possible need for additional interventions.

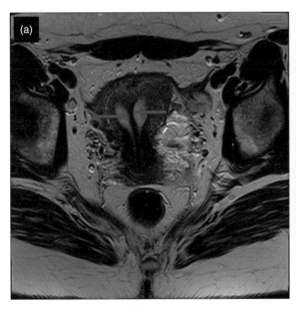
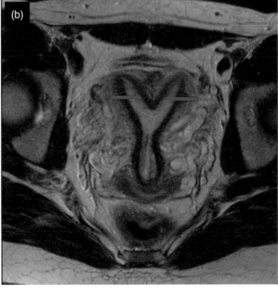

Figure 3B.7 MRI Septate Uterus
Transverse T2-weighted (a and b) scans of the pelvis
In the first image, there is a complete uterine septum that extended through the entire uterus and into the cervix. The septum (arrowed, a) is low signal and relatively thin, and this is fibrous and suitable for resection. In the second image, the septum is incomplete (arrowed, b) but is muscular and has the same imaging appearances as the myometrium. This septum would not be suitable for surgical resection.

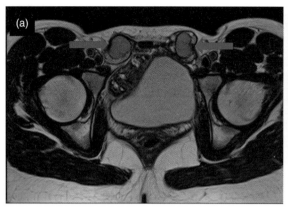
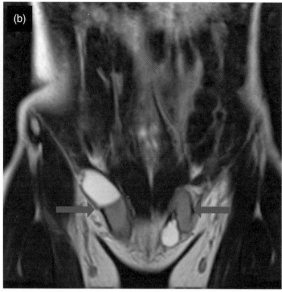

Figure 3B.8 MRI Complete Androgen Insufficiency Syndrome
Transverse T2-weighted (a) and coronal T2 weighted MRI (b) scans of the pelvis
There are bilateral inguinal testes in this patient with CAIS (arrowed, a and b). The testes are of intermediate signal on these images and above the right and below the left testis there are bight para-gonadal cysts, which are commonly seen in CAIS.

Androgen Insensitivity Syndrome

In Androgen Insensitivity Syndrome, the main function of imaging is to locate the testes (Figure 3B.8), assess them for malignancy, and if present, stage malignant disease. Testes can occur anywhere from the level of the kidney to the labia but are most commonly either in the groin, or in the pelvis. MRI can measure vaginal length.

Ultrasound has been shown to be a sensitive tool for identifying gonads within or caudal to the inguinal ring; however, for the identification of impalpable or intra-abdominal gonads [7], MRI is often better. On MRI, these gonads (Figure 3B.8) are usually slightly oval in shape, and they may be either homogeneous or heterogeneous, containing several low-signal nodules that correspond to Sertoli adenomas. They often have a distal, low-signal cap-like structure that is the pampiniform plexus. The testes are frequently associated with para-testicular cysts, which may vary in number and size.

Mayer-Rokitansky-Kuster-Hauser Syndrome

The diagnosis of Mayer-Rokitansky-Kuster-Hauser (MRKH) syndrome relies on the absence of a normal midline uterus and upper vagina. Rudimentary uteri

are found in MR scans in more than 90 percent of patients with MRKH [8], corresponding well with the best laparoscopic data, and these are almost invariably found at the inferior margin of the ovaries (Figure 3B.9). The uterine buds can vary in size from a few ml, up to around 80 ml [8]. They can be undifferentiated or show layers of differentiation. Some contain blood if the endometrium is functional, and some show features of adenomyosis; both of these conditions can be associated with pelvic pain. Uterine buds are characterized by an absence of a cervix, even in the most well developed.

Although a diagnosis of MRKH can be made with ultrasound, small rudimentary uterine buds and ectopic ovaries are not always visualized. The identification of the uterine buds is more reliable with MRI than ultrasound, and this finding confirms the diagnosis. A firm diagnosis can be helpful in directing appropriate care such as psychological support and also guidance on future fertility. Imaging can also be helpful in showing other associated anomalies, in particular the absence of a kidney in around 10 percent of cases [6]. MRI is useful for measuring vaginal length.

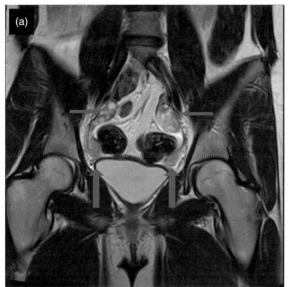 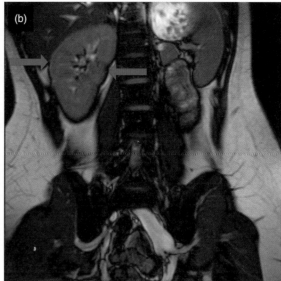

Figure 3B.9 MRI Mayer-Rokitansky-Kuser-Hauser Syndrome
Coronal T2-weighted (a and b) scans of the pelvis
Two adnexal ovaries are seen in this patient with MRKH syndrome (horizontal arrows, a). Below each ovary are small soft tissue nodules (vertical arrows, a), which are the rudimentary uteri. In this case the uterine buds are homogeneous and are not differentiated into layers.

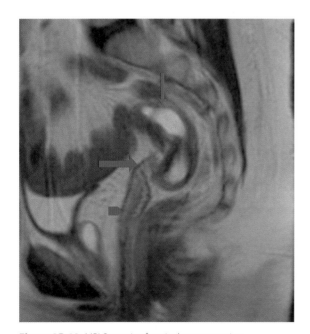

Figure 3B.10 MRI Stenosis of vaginal reconstruction
Sagittal T2-weighted scan of the pelvis
The midline uterus is distended by high-signal fluid (vertical arrow), due to stenosis (horizontal arrow) of the anastomosis of an intestinal neo-vagina (arrowhead) with the cervix.

Postoperative Assessment

MRI is often used to assess the complex postoperative pelvis in patients with Mullerian or cloacal anomalies who may present with secondary amenorrhea or recurrent pelvic pain. These patients may have undergone extensive urological and bowel surgery and have stomata and unpredictable anatomy due to the extensive reconstructive surgery. The function of imaging is to define the anatomy, and the complications of the anomaly and surgery such as hydrosalpinx, cysts, fistulae, and patency of reconstructed vaginas. Stenosis and obstruction of a reconstructed vagina (Figure 3B.10) or cervix may be a cause of recurrent pelvic pain. Incomplete resection of a rudimentary unicornuate uterus can result in restenosis and re-accumulation of blood products. Further, showing a "normal" postoperative pelvis can be reassuring and help direct other investigative and treatment options.

Classification of Congenital Mullerian Anomalies

Several systems are used to classify congenital Mullerian anomalies [9–12]. They have different strengths and weaknesses; however, in clinical practice the American

Society of Reproductive Medicine classification is commonly used [9]. The advantages of this system are its simplicity so it is easy to remember, it is widely used, and the abnormalities described relate to the embryology and help predict the need for surgery. The disadvantages are that it is incomplete and has limited application for detailed embryological research. However, when imaging patients, having a complete description of the abnormalities present largely offsets these deficiencies. Reports need to detail the structure, size, and extent of anomalies and complications present. This is also supplemented by close working team relationships and multidisciplinary meetings, which facilitate understanding of the anomalies and the patients themselves.

Conclusion and Future Developments

Ultrasound and MRI are non-ionizing, safe, and accurate imaging tools that help inform the diagnosis and management of children and adolescents with gynecological abnormalities. They are well-established imaging modalities with ultrasound used as the first-line modality and supplemented by MRI when necessary. The technology of both techniques is constantly improving; three-dimensional 3D imaging is becoming more common and of better quality. Assessment of uterine motility is another area of future development that may be useful for assessing uterine function and predicting likelihood of fertility.

References

1. Timor-Tritsch IE, Monteagudo A, Rebarber A et al. Transrectal scanning: an alternative when transvaginal scanning is not feasible. *Ultrasound Obstet Gynecol.* 2003; **21**(5): 473–79.

2. Rosenberg HK Sonography of the pelvis in patients with primary amenorrhea. *Endocrinol Metab Clin N Am* 2009; **38**: 739–60.

3. Cohen HL, Eisenberg P, Mandel F et al. Ovarian cysts are common in premenarchal girls: a sonographic study of 101 children 2–12 years old. *Am J Roentgenol* 1992; **159**: 89–91.

4. Humphries PD, Simpson JC, Creighton SM et al. MRI in the assessment of congenital vaginal anomalies. *Clin Radiol* 2008; **63**: 442–48.

5. Chang HC, Bhatt S, Dogra VS Pearls and pitfalls in diagnosis of ovarian torsion. *Radiographics.* 2008; **28**(5): 1355–68.

6. Hall-Craggs MA, Kirkham A, Creighton SM Renal and urological abnormalities occurring with Mullerian anomalies. *J Pediatr Urol.* 2013; **9**(1): 27–32.

7. Kanemoto K, Hayashi Y, Kojima Y et al. Accuracy of ultrasonography and magnetic resonance imaging in the diagnosis of non-palpable testis. *International Journal of Urology* 2005; **12**: 668–72.

8. Hall-Craggs MA, Williams CE, Pattison SH et al. Magnetic Resonance Imaging (MRI) in the diagnosis of Mayer-Rokitansky-Kuster-Hauser Syndrome. *Radiology* 2013; **269**: 787–92.

9. The American Fertility Society classifications of adnexal adhesions, distal tubal obstruction, tubal occlusions secondary to tubal ligation, tubal pregnancies, Müllerian anomalies and intrauterine adhesions. *Fertil Steril* 1998; **49**: 944–55.

10. Acien P, Acien M, Sanchez-Ferrer M Complex malformations of the female genital tract. New types and revision of classification. *Human Reproduction* 2004; **19**: 2377–84.

11. Oppelt P, Renner SP, Brucker S et al. The VCUAM (Vagina Cervix Uterus Adnex-assicuated Malformation) Classification: A new classification for genital malformations. *Fertility and Sterility* 2005; **84**: 1493–97.

12. Grimbizis GF, Gordts S, Di Spiezio Sardo A et al. The ESHRE/ESGE consensus on the classification of female genital tract congenital anomalies. *Human Reproduction* 2013; **28**: 2031–44.

Safeguarding for Pediatric and Adolescent Gynecology

Sveta Alladi and Deborah Hodes

Introduction and Definitions

Child maltreatment is a global issue that can affect children and young people in any setting and has short and long term impacts on their mental and physical health as well as their education attainment, social skills, and economic or employment potential. It is defined as follows:

> All forms of physical and/or emotional ill-treatment, sexual abuse, neglect or negligent treatment or commercial or other exploitation, resulting in actual or potential harm to the child's health, survival, development or dignity in the context of a relationship of responsibility, trust or power. [1]

The international community universally condemns child maltreatment. Currently 195 countries (all except the United States and South Sudan [2]) have ratified the United Nations Convention of the Rights of the Child (UNCRC). The treaty provides *protections* against exploitations, such as child abuse, reflected in Article 19, which states [3]: "All children have a right to protection from all forms of physical and mental violence, injury or abuse, neglect and maltreatment or exploitation, including sexual abuse while in the care of parent(s), legal guardians or another person who has the care of the child."

The World Health Organization (WHO) classifies most forms of child maltreatment into four main categories of abuse: physical, which includes fabricated illness and female genital mutilation (FGM); emotional or psychological; sexual; and neglect. A more expanded definition of child maltreatment now includes a fifth category of childhood sexual exploitation (CSE). In addition, trafficking, honor killings, forced marriage, online sexual abuse, and slavery are now recognized as forms of abuse.

Child Maltreatment – a Global Issue

Estimates of prevalence and incidence vary widely, depending on the country and the method of research used, particularly as there are no standardized statistics. In the United Kingdom, the National Society for the Prevention of Cruelty to Children (NSPCC) estimated that more than 57,000 children were in need of child protection services in 2015. In 2014, there were 42 deaths by assault or undetermined intent of children age 28 days to 14 years in the UK and 62 cases of homicide [4].

UNICEF estimates that violence took the lives of around 54,000 adolescent girls between the ages of 10 and 19, in 2012, making it the second leading cause of death among this population (Figure 4.1) [5].

The global community has addressed the issues in one of the sustainable development goals launched in January 2016, which outline the global priorities for the next 15 years. Goal 5, the goal for gender equality, outlines an aspiration to eliminate all forms of violence against women and girls such as trafficking and exploitation as well as harmful practices such as forced marriage and FGM.

Child Maltreatment – Why It Is Important

Gynecologists are in a unique position to recognize the signs and symptoms of child abuse at different times during the patient's management. Talking to a patient confidentially gives the child or young person the opportunity to disclose maltreatment. It is a recognized professional duty to identify and report child abuse in most industrialized nations; there is a mandatory duty to report child abuse in some states in the United States, Canada, Australia, Brazil, South Africa, and states in the European Union including Sweden.

Studies have shown that children who experience maltreatment are also at increased risk of short and long term physical and mental health conditions that include the following:

Unintended pregnancy, sexual transmitted diseases, sexual exploitation

Physical injury, for example, broken limbs, abusive head trauma resulting in death

Percentage distribution of deaths among **boys** aged 0 to 19 years in 2012, by cause and by age group

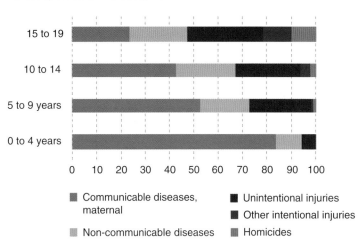

Communicable diseases, maternal

Non-communicable diseases

Unintentional injuries

Other intentional injuries

Homicides

Figure 4.1 Hidden in Plain Sight: A statistical analysis of violence against children, UNICEF, New York, 2014.
Source: World Health Organization, *Global Health Estimates (GHE) Summary Tables: Deaths by cause, age, sex and region, 2012*, WHO, Geneva, 2014, recalculated by UNICEF.

Percentage distribution of deaths among **girls** aged 0 to 19 years in 2012, by cause and by age group

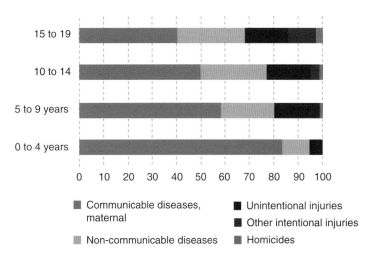

Communicable diseases, maternal

Non-communicable diseases

Unintentional injuries

Other intentional injuries

Homicides

Psychological effects, for example, depression, posttraumatic stress disorder, anxiety

Behavioral effects, for example, smoking, drug and alcohol misuse

Chronic disease, for example, heart disease, high blood pressure, and cancer

Poor early development, academic achievement, and social-emotional well-being

There are also societal consequences of child maltreatment. In the United States, abuse and neglect increase the likelihood of adult criminal behavior by 28 percent and violent crime by 30 percent [6]. Victims of abuse are also more likely to perpetuate the abuse cycle.

Recognizing Child Maltreatment and the Duty of the Pediatric and Adolescent Gynecologist

It is important that gynecologists have a clear idea of how to refer to local services when there is a suspicion or allegation of maltreatment. All areas will have local and national guidelines. Clinicians should also be up to date with basic training as suggested by their professional bodies.

A girl or young woman who is a victim of maltreatment may present in the outpatient clinic, when an in-patient, or in the emergency department (see Box 4.1)

BOX 4.1 Presentations of Child Abuse and Neglect to the Gynecologist

Allegation

Patient alleges abuse and or neglect, acute and/or historic sexual assault

Symptoms

Physical e.g. discharge, sorenes, bleeding medically unexplained symptoms

Signs

- Bruise unexplained, unusual position
- Bites
- Unexplained skin marks, burns etc
- Pregnant - unknown father, concealed, after rape
- Unkempt, dirty, or glamorous, that is, out of proportion to expectation, for example, looked-after child with expensive jewelry

Behavior child/YP

Clingy or withdrawn, going out more if a teenager frightened, not speaking and allowing parent or "boyfriend" to do so

Behavior of Parent

- Delays treatment of any condition especially serious conditions
- Noncompliance with treatment/failure to attend appointments
- Requesting unnecessary investigations and treatment

with a symptom and/or sign that may lead to a suspicion of maltreatment or there maybe a disclosure of an incidence of maltreatment including rape or exploitation. Remember to create an opportunity to speak to the child/young person alone. One way of doing this would be to say, "It is my usual practice to speak to children/young people on their own as part of my assessment."

If another doctor is present, such as a trainee, then it is often less threatening to suggest one sees the parent while the other the child but in different rooms.

It is important to recognize that

1. Several forms of abuse may coexist, for example, witnessing domestic violence and being subject to physical abuse and neglect.
2. There maybe abuse in addition to the underlying condition being treated, for example, emotional abuse and intersex.
3. There may be other coexisting diagnoses, e.g. sexual abuse and lichen sclerosis.

4. There is often a distinctive cultural context, for example, corporal punishment or FGM [7].

Remember that it is not only the younger child who is vulnerable. The developmental trajectory of adolescents who are living in a wide social context gives many opportunities for harm [8]. They are vulnerable to

1. Continuing maltreatment from childhood
2. Sexual exploitation
3. Cyberbullying
4. Gangs and peer-on-peer abuse
5. Forced marriage
6. Intimate partner violence

Health care practitioners are often concerned about how to approach the topic of maltreatment with the family and are worried about provoking a negative or angry response from parents. some patients presenting to gynecologists will be suffering some form of maltreatment, so despite these fears ensure that the well-being of the child/young person is paramount [9].

If there is suspicion of maltreatment, refer to the professional with expertise in child protection. This might be a pediatric doctor or specialist nurse. In the UK, a named doctor or nurse is available for safeguarding who is available to discuss cases and offer advice [10]. In the United States, similarly the hospital may have a specialist child protection team or specialist doctor. In the United States, there is also a mandatory duty to report to child protective services and the Child Advocacy Center [11]. A child protection specialist will undertake a more comprehensive assessment. You can explain your concerns to the family as follows: "I would like to get to the bottom of what is going on with your child and so will refer to my pediatric colleagues for support." If at any point there are concerns that the child is in an unsafe home environment, alert social services and if there is immediate danger the police.

Risk Factors in the Background History – Family and Social History

It is helpful to consider *protective* factors, which includes the child's resilience (ability to overcome adversity), and *vulnerability* factors to understand why a particular child is susceptible to abuse, all of which may be elicited during the history. A helpful statement to use is, "It is my usual practice/local policy to ask all families a number of questions about their background to help me with the assessment."

Despite challenging circumstances, parents may still have the capacity to give adequate care; for

33

BOX 4.2 Key Vulnerability Factors that may increase the suspicion of Child Maltreatment

Individual Factors

Parent

- Drug and alcohol misuse*
- Mental health concerns*
- Learning difficulties
- Chronic ill health
- Involved in criminal activity
- Unemployed or lack of financial support
- History of abuse or neglect

Child

- Learning difficulties/disability
- High medical need
- Mental ill health
- Result of an unwanted pregnancy
- Premature

Relationship Factors

- Parent and child failure to bond
- Domestic violence now called intimate partner violence between child's parents or caregivers*
- Parent is socially isolated
- Parent does not have support for parenting from extended family

Community Factors

- Lack of adequate housing
- Poverty
- Lack of services to support families in need
- Strong cultural beliefs leading to FGM, honor killing, child marriage, forced marriage
- Member of a gang
- Lack of educational opportunities

Further Social History

- Who is responsible for the care of the child? Who is the child ever alone with?
- Is the child attending school regularly? Has the school noticed any unusual behavior?
- Is the family known currently or in the past to social services? Have there been any previous allegations of abuse?
- Who is in the family? Where do they live and are they employed?
- Who is in the household (boyfriend, etc.)?

* These three together are known as the toxic trio being commonly found in the families of severely maltreated victims.

example, a mother with moderate depression may still be an excellent parent who prioritizes her child's needs. Therefore questions relating to a family's background should be approached sensitively and without judgment. Box 4.2 highlights some of the important factors to consider when child maltreatment is suspected.

Documentation

It is vital to keep clear, concise, and contemporaneous notes. These may be required for reports including witness statements for legal proceedings. Include the date, time, location, and persons present for each part of the consultation and who gave the history. Label body maps and diagrams to illustrate the location, dimensions, color, and texture of any marks identified on the skin, including birthmarks, as well as scars or bruising. Document, if known, with the cause of any marks and supplement with photographs if possible although the forensic examiner will usually do this.

A distinction should be made between observations and suspicions and interpretations in the notes. Where possible, it is useful to note down illustrative quotes, for example, "Mom always hits me on my back so my teacher can't see the marks."

Examination

If possible, extend the usual gynecological examination if there is a suspicion of maltreatment. This enables clear onward referral to the specialist. Include the following if possible:

– Height, weight, head circumference plotted on growth charts. (The child who is underweight or has stunted growth may lead to consideration or suspicion of neglect.)
– General appearance: Is the child wearing clean appropriate clothing? Is there any dirt under the nails? Has the hair been washed?
– General demeanor: Is the child withdrawn or scared? How is his or her interaction with the carer? Was the child cooperative?
– Whole-body examination of skin, hair, mouth, teeth, nose, head, and scalp. Hidden areas such as the neck, back of ears, soles of feet should also be examined.

– Systemic examination of cardiovascular, respiratory, and abdominal systems and other systems as indicated.
– Pubertal stage.
– Developmental milestones, cognitive ability – suspicion of learning difficulties: Did they follow your instructions? Did they understand your questions? Are they ambulant?
– Note if any part of the examination was omitted and if so why.

Physical Abuse

Physical abuse is defined as a form of abuse that may involve hitting, shaking, throwing, poisoning, burning or scalding, drowning, suffocating, or otherwise causing physical harm to a child. Fabricated or induced illness in a child by a parent or carer (FII), now understood as a spectrum, can be a form of physical abuse.

Recognizing a Child with Physical Abuse

It is common for children to have bruises on their skin particularly if they are ambulant or of school-going age (Figure 4.2). A child who is or has been the victim of physical abuse may or may not present with visible physical signs on examination. However, injuries such as bruising (Figure 4.3), scars, bites, or burns on examination may arouse suspicion of maltreatment. Other features that may arouse suspicion are listed in Box 4.3. Figures 4.2 and 4.3 are body maps showing patterns of accidental and abusive bruising [12].

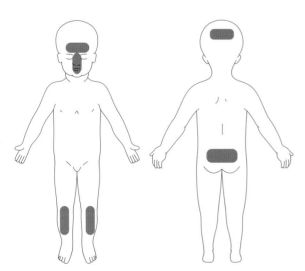

Figure 4.2 Body maps showing pattern of bruising in accidental injury

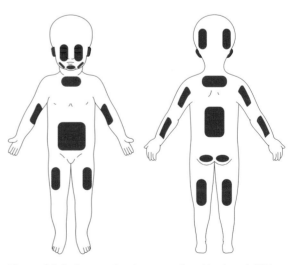

Figure 4.3 Body maps showing pattern found in abused children

> **BOX 4.3** Features That May Arouse Suspicion of Maltreatment
>
> – Unusual location of injury, for example, bruising behind ears or upper thighs
> – Skin marks suggestive of self-inflicted trauma in deliberate self-harm.
> – Injury in a nonambulant child
> – Delayed presentation of injury, for example, "I think she fell more than two days ago but I didn't have time to bring her to the doctor."
> – Inconsistent or changing story, for example, "She must have fallen over in school – actually her dad said he banged her leg in the kitchen."
> – Unclear mechanism of injury.
> – Abnormal interaction between carer and child, for example, child is withdrawn in presence of adult.
> – Aggressive or defensive behavior of carers toward each other or health care staff
> – Child gives other history/no history or gives the impression of being coached.

Investigations and further management of physical abuse

Fabricated or Induced Illness (FII, previously Munchausen's-by-Proxy)

Fabricated or induced illness is a rare form of child abuse, which usually falls under the category of physical abuse. Now it is considered a spectrum, from an anxious or mentally unwell parent, usually the mother, exaggerating symptoms in the child, to the abusive parent who fabricates or induces illness e.g. the mother who puts her own menstrual blood in her prepubertal child's underwear and presents her with vaginal bleeding

Managing this disorder presents as a challenge for the practitioner who needs to strike a balance between ruling out a true medical illness while avoiding over-investigation of symptoms. Reassuring the parent that there is no medical cause for symptoms may help but continuing support and review are often needed to stop further unnecessary investigations. The family may require referral to the multi-agency team –social services police.

Recognizing FII

The signs of FII include the following:

– High level of anxiety from parent/carer and requests for repeat consultations

– Parent requesting more investigations and treatment
– No cause identified for presenting features
– Exaggeration of symptoms, for example, profuse bleeding that is never observed
– Many opinions sought

You may suspect child maltreatment, if features as listed in Box 4.3 are present e.g. unexplained bruising on the the inner thighs. As part of the further management, explain to the mother that a second opinion from Pediatric colleagues is in the child's best interest.

As part of the complete assessment, investigations need to be arranged to rule out any medical causes of bruising or injury, such as Von Willebrand disease. Discuss with a hematologist if there is any family history of bleeding disorders.

First line investigations include

– Full blood count, white cell count, hemoglobin, and platelet
– Coagulation screen

Neglect

Neglect is defined as the persistent failure to meet a child's basic physical and/or psychological needs, likely to result in the serious impairment of the child's health or development.

Recognizing a Neglected Child

Neglect frequently coexists with other types of abuse. It is harmful and can be life threatening and needs to be taken as seriously as other forms of abuse. Some of the categories of neglect include

– Emotional neglect (emotional neglect is often described with emotional abuse) – inability to interact with child/young person appropriately.
– Abandonment – child found unattended in the home, missing from home, runaways.
– Medical neglect – missed clinic appointments, poor dentition.
– Nutritional neglect – inadequate growth.
– Educational neglect – poor school attendance, truanting.
– Physical neglect – unkempt and dirty appearance.
– Failure to provide supervision – recurrent accidents, sexual exploitation.

CASE EXAMPLE 4.A

Joanna is a Caucasian 10-year-old girl with recurrent pelvic pain. She attends with her mother who has a history of depression. Joanna appears withdrawn throughout the consultation.

What Questions Could Inform the Differential Diagnosis of Child Maltreatment?

– It would be appropriate to ask about the mother's mental health status. Is she on medication? Does she require inpatient treatment? Does the mother feel able to care for Joanna? Who else is caring for the child?
– Ask questions regarding domestic violence (Box 4.4).

Joanna's mother discloses that there has been domestic violence between her and her partner in the past. She states that Joanna has not witnessed any incidents. The family had been known to social services briefly in the past. Mother has not accessed any support recently.
However on routine physical examination there is extensive bruising on Joanna's inner thighs and abdomen.

Next Steps

– These are unusual places for a child to have bruising. Ask questions of mother and child regarding the mechanism of injury. For example, *how did Joanna get these marks?*
– If possible, speak to Joanna alone.
– Complete a thorough examination of Joanna's skin and all systems.
– Document clear and precise notes following the guidelines listed earlier. Ensure that the location, size, and type of mark are listed and the reported mechanism of injury.

Joanna denies that she has suffered any injuries but when seen alone says she doesn't like her mother's partner. Mother says Joanna must have fallen in the park. The explanations for the bruising are different and sexual abuse needs to be considered given the site of the bruises.

> **BOX 4.4** Domestic Violence – Questions
>
> – Who lives at home? How are things at home?
> – Has anyone at home hit you or tried to injure you in any way?
> – Are you afraid of your partner? Do you ever feel in danger?
> – Ask regarding past history of contact with social services or history of any type of abuse including sexual assault in both mother and child.

Emotional Abuse

Emotional abuse is defined as the persistent emotional maltreatment of a child such as to cause severe and persistent adverse effects on the child's emotional development; it is noticeable in the parent-child interaction.

Recognizing of Emotional Abuse

Emotional abuse and neglect are forms of psychological maltreatment of children and maybe seen as less serious than other forms of abuse and neglect because they have no immediate physical effects. However, persistent psychological maltreatment is associated with aggression, depression, and antisocial behavior later in life. This form of abuse is correlated with maternal depression. Some characteristics of the interaction between the child and caregiver or the child's behavior may indicate emotional abuse or neglect [13].

Observations of emotional abuse include
In the parent:

– Parent not being emotionally engaged with the child's needs.
– Parent describes baby as irritating and demanding.
– Parent/caregiver is unresponsive to the child/young person and fails to respond to appropriately.
– Parent/caregiver is critical or verbally aggressive and often has unrealistic expectations.
– No praise or positive reinforcement is given.

CASE EXAMPLE 4.B

A prepubertal 8-year-old girl, Jenny of African origin presents to the emergency department with a two-day history of vaginal bleeding.

What Questions Could Inform the Differential Diagnosis of Child Maltreatment?
Along with a thorough medical history, the girl and family should be asked about any history of trauma to the groin area, both accidental and inflicted from sexual abuse. Ask to see the underwear with the blood to try and establish if the bleeding is urethral, vaginal, or anal in origin.
There is no history of trauma preceding the vaginal bleeding. No family history of female genital mutilation (FGM). No past history of concerns regarding abuse. No other concerning factors were detected in the initial history. Take the opportunity to see the child alone to ask about self-inflicted trauma and sexual abuse.

Next Steps
The girl needs a full examination including anogenital examination. Initial investigations include urine tests to confirm hematuria and look for infection and blood tests to rule out precocious puberty and bleeding disorders.
The child is noted to have mild vulvovaginitis (no other findings – ulceration, anal fissures, etc. – which may explain the bleeding – see Chapter 6), which is treated and resolves on subsequent examinations.

Further presentations
However, Jenny presents frequently to the clinic. Her mother describes "cupfulls" of blood being lost with each episode and appears increasingly distressed. At each presentation, there is no medical cause for the bleeding described, no anemia detected in the child, and no underwear bought despite many requests. Jenny is always very quiet and says she doesn't know about the bleeding when asked.

Further Management
If there is no medical cause for the vaginal bleeding, consider fabricated illness in the differential diagnosis. Because of the challenging nature of diagnosis and management of FII, seek support from a pediatric specialist. Support the diagnostic progress by compiling a chronology of symptoms, presentations, and investigations. A balance needs to be struck between excessive investigations of unexplained symptoms and addressing the anxiety of the parent.

In the child:

– Overly affectionate toward strangers.
– Lacks confidence or becomes wary or anxious.
– Does not have close relationship with parent.
– Aggressive toward others/poor social skills.

In the adolescent:

– Risky behaviors.
– Depression and anxiety.
– Unexpected manner and language for age.
– Struggles to control strong emotions or has extreme outbursts.
– Seems isolated from parents.
– Lacks social skills or has few, if any, friends.
– Missing, truanting from school.
– Signs of deliberate self-harm.

Childhood Sexual Abuse (CSA)

Childhood sexual abuse (CSA) may be acute or nonacute and involves forcing or enticing a child or young person to take part in sexual activities, including prostitution, whether or not the child is aware of what is happening. The activities may involve physical contact, including penetrative (e.g., rape, sodomy, or oral sex) or non-penetrative acts. They may include non-contact activities, such as involving children in looking at, or in the production of, sexual online images, watching sexual activities, or encouraging children to behave in sexually inappropriate ways.

Recognizing of Sexual Abuse

Evidence suggests that a large proportion of girls who have been sexually abused in childhood often disclose months or years later, including in adulthood [14]. Sometimes they present later with chronic pelvic pain. So if an empathetic listener asks about a history of sexual abuse either acute or historic, then the girl may reveal her history. CSA may be the result of intra- or extra-familial abuse, with the former more common. In the majority of cases, the perpetrator is likely to be a male member of the family, including the father, stepfather, mother's boyfriend, and older brother [15].

CASE EXAMPLE 4.C

A 2-year-old South Asian child with ambiguous genitalia noted at birth presents to a follow-up clinic. She attends with both parents. She is noted to be underweight and appears upset.

What Questions Could Inform the Differential Diagnosis of Child Maltreatment?

– How is the family dealing with the diagnosis? Do the parents need counseling or emotional support?
– What is the family's cultural background? How has the community responded to the diagnosis? Ask questions around FGM. (See later in chapter.)
– Who is responsible for caring for the child? How is the mother's interaction with the child? Does the family have extended family support?
– What is the child's diet? Has the child always been underweight?

The parents describe they have found it difficult to deal with the diagnosis. They had been expecting a male child. The extended family has ostracized them and so they are socially isolated. The mother is finding it difficult to bond with the child. The weight of the child has been dropping from the 50th centile at 1 year and is now on the 0.4th centile.

Next Steps

– The emotional status of the mother and social isolation of the family should lead to a consideration of child maltreatment.
– It is worrying that the child's weight is dropping. Consider neglect as part of the differential diagnosis and consider other forms of maltreatment that may coexist.

Other observations include the child has soiled clothes and dirt under her fingernails; the mother appears passive and does not seem to respond when the child is tearful during the examination.

Investigations and Management

When there is a suspicion of neglect, as with any other form of child maltreatment, complete a full assessment including ruling out any medical causes for the presentation. Refer to a pediatrician to assist you with further investigations and management, for example, coexisting malabsorption.

In addition, consider referring the family for psychological support and to social services for further investigations.

Intra-familial abuse often follows a pattern, starting with a period of grooming by the perpetrator. This may include exposure to pornography, inappropriate touching, and digital penetration and then progresses to anal, oral, or vaginal penetration. The victim may be emotionally manipulated over months or years with threats and bribes. These young women may not disclose because they fear they will not be believed or feel guilty about the consequences for the family. As such, when they do present it is frequently non-acute and there may not be any physical signs on examination. Sexual exploitation, which includes peer-on-peer abuse, is increasingly recognized [16].

Management of Acute Sexual Assault

A young girl or woman, less often a prepubertal girl may present following an acute sexual assault or rape. If she presents within the time frame for collection of forensic evidence, then referral to the local center is urgent. Ensure referral details are available and refer without delay; it will usually be to a child advocacy center (United States) or the SARC – Sexual Assault Referral Centre (UK).

Ideally, forensic evidence is collected within 12 hours of the alleged assault (Table 4.1). The maximum time recommended between the assault and examination is as follows:

Table 4.1 Time limits for detection of spermatozoa and seminal fluids

Site	Spermatozoa	Seminal Fluid
Vagina	6 days	12–18 hours
Anus	3 days	3 hours
Mouth	12–14 hours	–
Clothing/bedding	Until washed	Until washed

BOX 4.5 Physical Genital Signs of Acute Sexual Assault/Rape

Genital Signs

- Genital erythema
- Genital edema
- Genital bruising
- Genital abrasions
- Lacerations to hymen, posterior forchette, and fossa navicularis

Anal Signs

- Anal tears, abrasions, or bruising
- Anal lacerations – exclude inflammatory bowel disease and constipation (penetration from within – large stool may cause anal fissure)

Later Signs

- Transection of hymen
- Deep notch of hymen

Within three days for girls younger than age 13 (prepubertal)

Within seven days for girls older than age 13 (pubertal)

Physical injuries maybe seen and photographed within a three-week time frame

See Box 4.5 for the physical signs that may be found after sexual assault both acutely and later

Recognizing of CSA

A girl or young woman may present in a number of ways with a history of having been groomed, sexually abused and/or raped:

- Allegation by the child, sibling, parent, or carer
- Behavioral or emotional difficulties, for example, inappropriate sexualized behaviors
- Physical symptoms, such as secondary enuresis, encopresis and smearing, headaches, and gastrointestinal disturbances (e.g., recurrent abdominal pain)
- Physical signs on anogenital examination, which are rare (see Box 4.5)
- Sexually transmitted infections – gonorrhea, chlamydia, genital herpes, or any of the blood-borne viruses especially in children younger than age 13
- Unexplained, concealed pregnancy

CASE EXAMPLE 4.D

Helen, a 5-year-old girl presents with a five-week history of increasing thick, white vaginal discharge.

What Questions Could Inform the Differential Diagnosis of Child Maltreatment?

Ask Helen what she calls her genitalia and anus and use this term during the consultation (Table 4.2) [17]. Has the child had any other unexplained new symptoms, for example, soiling or incontinence? Ask about the home environment and who lives at home. Ask about the child's behavior. Has there been a change in behavior? Does the child display any unusual behaviors (e.g., sexualized behavior)?

Helen is any only child. She lives with her mother and her mother's new partner of 3 months. The new partner is responsible for Helen's care in the evening before Helen's mother comes home from work. For the past 6 weeks, Helen has displayed more challenging behavior.

Table 4.2 Some terms used by young girls for female genitalia

Bum
Couchie
Fan fan
Flower
Minnie
Pee pee
Pumpum
Tuttut
Winkie

Next Steps

Given the suspicions, take a swab for culture and sensitivity. In addition, the history of behavior change and home circumstance may add to a suspicion of child maltreatment. However, vulvovaginitis is common in the prepubertal child (see Chapter 6) but could also be associated with maltreatment.

Take the opportunity to ask the child who is allowed to look at or touch her genitalia and who she should tell if she is worried. Advise the child how to act if anyone tries to touch her inappropriately – she has the right to say no. The NSPCC in the UK has an "Underwear Rule" campaign with accompanying resources for parents and children available to share with the family [18].

The microbiology laboratory results indicate that the vaginal swab is growing gonorrhea, which is highly suspicious for sexual abuse in a 5-year-old child.

Further management

Do Not Treat But Refer Urgently to the Specialist for Forensic Examination

The child requires a full physical examination including of the anogenital area. This is best done by the pediatric forensic examiner with the skills and competences to do so and the use of the colposcope for magnification and photo documentation. Guidelines for such examinations need to be followed, including screening for all sexually transmitted infections as well as confirming the gonorrhea, which must be sent with a chain of evidence form, storage of intimate images, written reports for social services and the court, and ability to act as a witness in court. See Royal College of Pediatrics and Child Health (RCPCH) and the American Association of Pediatrics (AAP) guidelines [19,20,21].

Further history and discussion with social services reveals that the mother's boyfriend is a sex offender.

Childhood Sexual Exploitation

Childhood sexual exploitation (CSE) is an insidious and hidden form of sexual abuse. The child or young person is placed in an exploitative situation or relationship where he or she may receive gifts, affection, food, as well as drugs and alcohol, in exchange for performing sexual acts or having sexual acts performed on him or her. In many cases the young person may not be aware that the exploitation is even taking place or may feel powerless to speak up about the abuse.

CSE does not always require physical contact. Increasingly, such abuse takes place online; a young person may be asked to send sexually explicit images or videos, via text message, email, or social media. The abuser may share these images widely as well as threatening to share them with others known to the child as a form of manipulation. It also occurs in gangs as a tool to exert power over other members, initiate members into the gang, or gain status within the gang.

There is not much information available as to the prevalence and circumstances of CSE globally. A UK-based study suggests that the majority of perpetrators are male and range in age from 12 to 75 [16].

It may be difficult to recognize children who are victims of CSE, as they may display no signs or symptoms at all. However there are some alerting features in the history:

- A recent change in behavior, for example, hostility toward parents, increased secrecy, displaying mood swings
- Recurrent sexually transmitted infections (STIs)
- Low self-esteem and/or evidence of self-harm
- Losing contact with peers and associating with an older age group
- Excessive and secret use of the internet and social media
- Receiving unexplained expensive gifts
- Alcohol or substance misuse
- Going missing overnight or frequently arriving home late

Box 4.6 gives a list of questions to ask a young person if suspicions are raised [21] (see also case example 4E).

Female Genital Mutilation (FGM)

FGM is a traditional and cultural practice, which WHO defines as procedures that remove or damage the external female genital organs for no medical reason (see Box 6.7 for types of FGM). FGM has no known health benefits. It is a violation of human rights, regarded as a form of child abuse and is an illegal practice in many countries around the world including the UK, United States, Australia, and France. The United Nations International Children's Emergency Fund (UNICEF) suggests that at least 200 million girls have been subjected to the practice, which may have physical and psychological sequelae [22]. A large proportion of FGM is thought to occur in African countries; more than 90 percent of girls and women (ages 5–49) in Guinea, Djibouti, and Somalia have undergone this practice. Now there is evidence of the practice in other countries such as Yemen, Malaysia, and Indonesia.

FGM is not mandated by any religious scriptures, although practitioners of FGM may misinform individuals that it is a necessary religious practice. Other

---

CASE EXAMPLE 4.E

A 14-year-old presents with an unwanted pregnancy. Her mother is extremely concerned as the girl has been moody lately and secretive about her whereabouts. The mother suspects the father of the child is an older boy who has recently been arrested for stabbing someone in the street.

BOX 4.6 Sexual Relationships (Questions for an Older Child/Adolescent)

- Are you having sexual relations with anyone?
- If no, when was the last time you did? If yes, are you happy with the person you are having sex with?
- How old is the person you are having sex with?
- How many people have you had sex with in the past 3 months? 12 months?
- Where did you meet the person you have sex with? Where do you spend time?
- Do you feel you could say no to sex?
- Have you ever been made to feel scared or uncomfortable by the person/s you have been having sexual contact with?
- Have you ever been made to do something sexual that you didn't want to do, or been intimidated?
- Has anyone ever given you something like gifts, money, drugs, alcohol or protection for sex?
- Have you ever been involved in sending or receiving messages of a sexual nature? Does anyone have pictures of you of a sexual nature? [21]

BOX 4.8 FGM Questions

- There are some communities that traditionally practice "cutting" or "circumcision." (If appropriate use term in patients' local language.) Are you from such a community?
- Does your family practice cutting or FGM? Have you considered FGM for your child? Or if older child, have you had FGM?

justifications may include preparation of a girl for marriage, ensuring chastity, or reducing libido [23].

Recognition of FGM

At time of writing, no child or young person has yet presented acutely after an FGM procedure in the UK. Such presentations would include hemorrhage, pain, urinary retention, wound infection, and sepsis.

The child or young person may present to the gynecology clinic with chronic symptoms as a consequence of FGM. These may include slow urinary flow and painful menstruation the later usually unrelated to the procedure. More likely FGM may be an incidental finding when:

1. Taking a history for contraception advice
2. Examining a young girl's genitalia
3. Performing a termination of pregnancy

BOX 4.7 World Health Organization (WHO) Classification of FGM

Type 1: Clitoridectomy: partial or total removal of the clitoris (a small sensitive and erectile part of the female genitals) and in rare cases only the prepuce (the fold of skin surrounding the clitoris).

Type 2: Excision: partial or total removal of the clitoris and labia minora with or without removal of the labia majora (the labia are "the lips" that surround the vagina).

Type 3: Infibulation: narrowing of the vaginal opening through the creation of a covering seal. The seal is formed by cutting and repositioning the labia minora or majora with or without removal of the clitoris.

Type 4: Other: all other harmful procedures to the genital for nonmedical reasons, for example, pricking, piercing, incision, scraping, and cauterizing the genital area. [24]

Asking about FGM should be routine in every consultation. Box 4.8 provides statements that can be used to introduce the topic with the family.

Forced or Early Child Marriage

Another significant issue, and human rights violation, affecting many young women globally is the practice of forced or early child marriage [25]. It is predicted that 142 million girls are likely to be married by their 18th birthday over the next decade. It predominately occurs in developing countries; 52 countries have a child marriage prevalence of greater than 25 percent. Child marriage puts young girls at higher risk of early pregnancy and its associated complications, STIs, as well as mental health complications such as depression. In forced marriages, a young girl who has been sexually active may present for hymenal reconstruction.

Following are a few screening questions that may be helpful:

- Do you think your parents have plans for your marriage?
- Have you ever been married or lived together with a man as if married?
- How old were you when you first started living with him?
- Did you feel like you could say no to living with/marrying this man?

CASE EXAMPLE 4.F

A 15-year-old girl from Eritrea is referred to the clinic from the primary care provider with a history of painful urination and painful menstruation since menarche at age 11.

What Questions Could Inform the Differential Diagnosis of Child Maltreatment?

In addition to the questions in Box 4.8, determine if the mother or other female family members have had FGM, particularly any younger or older sisters. On examination of the girl's genitalia, there is significant scarring (Figure 4.4). This is Type 3 FGM, the most severe form of FGM and could explain this young girl's symptoms.

Next Steps

FGM has medical and psychological consequences. Both need to be addressed. In Type 3 FGM, as in this case, a deinfibulation procedure can be offered to divide any scar tissue. Consider a referral for counseling services to support the young woman who may be emotionally affected from the trauma of FGM.

The family should be told that FGM is an illegal practice and informed of the law and that a referral to police and social services is mandatory in the UK and some states in the United States.

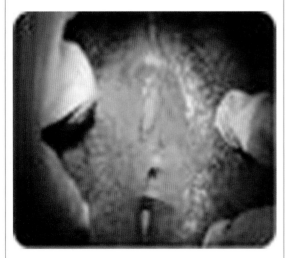

Figure 4.4 Type 3 Female Genital Mutilation

CASE EXAMPLE 4.G

A 6-year-old girl is referred for an examination for a suspicion of FGM. The girl had recently disclosed to her schoolteacher that her baby sister had FGM performed on a recent family trip to Malaysia.

On examination the genitalia appear abnormal. There is some mild scaring around the clitoral hood, which is consistent with Type 4 FGM (Figure 4.5).

Next Steps

Discuss the findings with the girl and her family and explain that there should not be any medical consequences. As the girl underwent the procedure at age 6 months, she would have no memory of it; but as an illegal practice, information needs to be shared with the multiagency team.

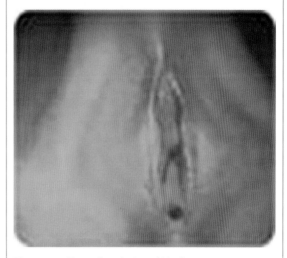

Figure 4.5 Type 4 Female Genital Mutilation

Gynecologists must be alert to the possibility of maltreatment of a child or young person presenting.

When appropriate, the pediatric gynecologist should ask key questions, perform a thorough examination, and refer as per their local guidelines seeking support from pediatric and child protection colleagues in their organization.

CSE, forced or early child marriage, and FGM are considered forms of child abuse. Practitioners should be aware of these issues and how to recognize children at risk.

Practitioners should involve parents in their enquiries, where it is safe to do so and escalate to the multiagency team when there is a concern. This may be urgent if a significant risk to the child's or young person's safety is determined.

Key Messages

Child maltreatment, in its various forms, is a human rights violation that affects children in large numbers globally.

References

1. Krug EG, Mercy D, Dahlber L et al. World report on violence and health. Geneva, World Health Organization, *Lancet* **360**.9339 (2002): 1083–88.

2. UN News – UN Lauds Somalia as Country Ratifies Landmark Children's Rights Treaty. *UN News Service Section*. N.p., 2016. Web June 27.

3. The United Nations Convention on the Rights of the Child. *Treaty Series* 1989; **1577**: 3.

4. Bentley H, O'Hagan O, Brown A et al. *How Safe Are Our Children? The Most Comprehensive Overview of Child Protection in the UK*. London: NSPCC, 2016.

5. Center for Disease Control Child Maltreatment. 2014. Print.

6. Widom CS, Maxfield MG *An Update on the Cycle of Violence*. Washington, DC: U.S. Department of Justice, Office of Justice, February 2001.

7. Raman S, Hodes D Cultural issues in child maltreatment. *Journal of Pediatrics and Child Health* **48**.1 (2011): 30–37. Web.

8. Khadr SN, Viner RM, Goddard A. Safeguarding in adolescence: under-recognised and poorly addressed. *Archives of Disease in Childhood* **96**.11 (2011): 991–94. Web.

9. Children Act 1989, London: HMSO.

10. HM Government Working Together to Safeguard Children: A Guide to Inter-Agency Working to Safeguard and Promote the Welfare of Children. 2015. Print.

11. Christian CW The evaluation of suspected child physical abuse. *Pediatrics*, **135**.5 (2015): e1337–e54. Web.

12 Maguire S Bruising as an indicator of child abuse: when should I be concerned? *Pediatrics and Child Health* **18**.12 (2008): 545–49 [Abstract from Science Direct].

13. Core Info. Parent-Child Interaction. Cardiff University, 2016. Web. May 13, 2016. Cardiff Child Protection Systematic Review.

14. Smith DW et al. Delay in disclosure of childhood rape: results from a national survey. *Child Abuse & Neglect* **24**.2 (2000): 273–87. Web.

15. Borg K, Snowdon C, Hodes D Child sexual abuse: recognition and response when there is a suspicion or allegation. *Pediatrics and Child Health* **24**.12 (2014): 536–43. Web.

16. Berelowitz S, Clifton J, Firimin C et al. If only someone had listened, London: Office of the Children's Commissioner (2013).

17. Scolnik D, Atkinson V, Hadi M et al. words used by children and their primary caregivers for private body parts and functions. *CMAJ: Canadian Medical Association Journal*, **169**.12 (2003): 1275–79.

18. The Underwear Rule. NSPCC. N.p., 2016. Web. May 13, 2016.

19. Royal College of Pediatrics and Child Health Physical signs of child sexual abuse: evidence-based review and guidance for best practice (2015).

20. www2.aap.org/sections/childabuseneglect/policies.cfm

21. Brook || *Spotting the Signs. CSE Proforma*. Brook.org. uk. N.p., 2016. Web. May 13, 2016.

22. UNICEF *Female Genital Mutilation/Cutting: A Global Concern*. UNICEF, 2016. www.unicef.org.

23. Creighton SM, Hodes D Female genital mutilation: what every paediatrician should know. *Archives of Disease in Childhood* (2015): archdischild-2014-307234. Web.

24. World Health Organization Classification of Female Genital Mutilation N.p., 2016. Web. June 27, 2016.

25. Glinski AM, Sexton M, Meyers L Sept. 2015. Washington DC: The Child, Early, and Forced Marriage Resource Guide Task Order, Banyan Global

Informed Consent in Pediatric and Adolescent Gynecology Practice: From Ethical Principles to Ethical Behaviors

Lih-Mei Liao, Paul M. Chadwick, and Anne Tamar-Mattis

In pediatric and adolescent gynecology (PAG), consent is required for a vast array of interventions ranging from commonplace procedures such as cystoscopy to controversial interventions such as labiaplasty. The process may be more or less involved according to the clinical scenario. A simple and low-risk procedure for clear medical reasons will require less discussion than an invasive intervention whose benefits and risks are disputed. A single blanket protocol to fit all clinical scenarios is therefore unacceptable [1].

Informed consent to elective and non-lifesaving medical interventions is the focus of this chapter. These situations are emblematic of dilemmatic decision making in conditions of uncertainty and highlights the influence of complex psychosocial factors. Social and psychological theories emphasize the individual, familial, cultural, and political contexts in which choices relating to health and illness are made. Some knowledge of the intra- and interpersonal processes can facilitate the translation of sound ethical principles into sound professional behaviors.

Nobel Prize winner Daniel Kahneman has deciphered decades of social psychological research to help us understand that much decision making is driven by cognitive shortcuts known as "heuristics" or "rules of thumb" that are influenced by, among other factors, how the information is framed and its emotional valence for the decision maker [2]. Heuristics are especially active under conditions of uncertainty and may be particularly influential in persons whose cognitive and emotional maturity is not yet optimal or who has had fewer opportunities to learn from the outcomes of previous treatment decisions.

The aim of this chapter is to provide practical solutions to address the gap between principles and practice of bioethics. The chapter begins by outlining the core principles, proceeds to discuss pertinent psychosocial variables that can impede implementation, and ends with practical ideas for improving informed consent.

Core Principles of Bioethics

Myriad clinical scenarios mean that formulas and templates for informed consent may always have limited applicability. However, the generic core principles cannot be compromised. In this section, the basic requirements are outlined, before considering the psychosocial barriers to their translation into clinical practice.

Beyond Legal Requirement

Legal standards generally require informing the patient of the diagnosis and prognosis; the procedure; the risks, benefits, and unknowns of any proposed treatment; and the risks, benefits, and unknowns of any available alternatives including no treatment. As much as possible, this information should be made specific to the individual for whom the treatment is proposed. A common way of stating the legal mandate in US jurisdictions, for example, is that physicians must provide the patient "as much information as [he/she] needs to make an informed decision, including any risk that a reasonable person would consider important in deciding to have the proposed treatment or procedure" [3].

However, informed consent is an ethical as well as a legal imperative, and ethical standards may go beyond bare legal requirements [4]. It is a well-accepted principle of bioethics that physicians have a responsibility to respect the autonomy of patients, including the patient's right to complete information when determining whether or not to undergo a proposed medical intervention. To give full informed consent, patients must be aware of their medical condition and able to weigh the risks and benefits of all possible options (including no treatment) to ensure that their decision reflects their personal goals and values [1].

Patients who feel appropriately involved in decision making have better outcomes, which makes it vital to allow flexibility and choice in how much patients are involved [5,6]. However, research suggests that more than one-third of patients are dissatisfied with the level of involvement in their care [5,7]. What complicates the situation is that the quantity of patient involvement is not static [8]. For example, in oncology, a patient may be happy for the clinician to make a decision based on "best practice" at the point of diagnosis, but within palliative care a patient may prefer more active involvement in decision making [9,10].

Patient Capacity

Children can participate in some medical decisions before they are old enough to provide legally valid consent to treatment. Younger children who can understand the basic aspects of an intervention can provide assent (informed agreement) for and may sometimes refuse treatment. By age 14, many children have the cognitive ability (if not the legal capacity) to make medical decisions [11]. Respect for children's developing autonomy requires involving them in medical decisions to the extent capable, which means explaining the most complex of treatments in terms that are developmentally relevant and can be understood, and respecting their right to refuse treatment when appropriate. It also requires practitioners to allow for progression toward children's greater involvement in their health care decisions as they develop, and it sometimes requires postponing elective procedures until the child matures.

Best Interest

Certain parental decisions may be culturally or religiously expedient but in the long term limit the child's open future, for instance, a child with a life-threatening need for a blood transfusion while the parents who are Jehovah's Witnesses prefer their child not to be transfused because of their religious beliefs [12]. Because the child is too immature to choose her own religion, she has a right to receive lifesaving interventions (even over parental objection) so that she can mature sufficiently to make her own religious decisions. As such, the child's right to an open future trumps the parents' right to raise their child as they wish.

The child's right to an open future requires clinicians and surrogates to balance the short- and long-term benefits and risks of all options. If the openness of the child's future is clearly enhanced by a particular option, which may include no treatment, then the deciding adults have an obligation to choose that option on behalf of the child, in the absence of an option that serves the child's best interest. As the child matures, she may choose from among the various options open to her. In some clinical situations this can be a highly complex, dilemmatic, and emotional process. Where the treatment option is not lifesaving, sufficient time and opportunities for discussion are crucial.

In situations where a surrogate, such as a parent, provides consent, respect for autonomy requires the decision makers to consider the perspective of the child's open future. Caregivers' preferences should not override the focus on the patient's best interest in the long term. While parents may make many medical decisions on behalf of their children, there are limits to parental authority in the medical context [11]. For example, parents in most US jurisdictions do not have authority to consent to elective sterilization of a child without court oversight [13]. Parents in many countries do not have the authority to consent to female genital cutting for social, religious, or cultural reasons even if carried out in a medical setting.

Barriers to the Implementation

The information given to patients or their surrogates is of central importance in ensuring that all three ethical principles – legal requirement, patient capacity, and best interests – are addressed and met. A range of psychosocial factors also needs addressing. These factors can impinge on decision dynamics in ways not always obvious; that is, they can subtly influence *what* [14] and *how* [15] information is shared with consequences for informed decision making.

Patient and Surrogate Factors

Emotion processing is integral to decision making; the recognition of this is implicit in the routine recommendation of a "cooling off" period before a decision is made. That is to say, health professionals are advised not to ask patients or surrogates to sign a written consent after a single discussion. Cancer specialists are perhaps the most adept at recognizing that treatment options are, more often than not, contemplated, discussed, and decided on in highly emotive contexts. Psychological research in cancer has demonstrated that people's recall of "bad news consultations" is often fragmented and not organized in a coherent narrative, at times with stark misconceptions about what was and was not said [16]. These observations are compatible with cognitive scientists' evidence that emotional arousal can alter our computation of probability and value [17]. Treatment decisions made suboptimal by overwhelming emotional distress is highly significant for informed consent.

Many clinical situations can trigger high emotions. One such example in PAG is the birth of a child with a genital difference. The shock of finding out the diagnosis and the fear of the child failing to develop socially acceptable gender and sexuality could have a number of effects. One of them may be a premature decision to opt into a surgical trajectory involving multiple operations and genital examinations without clear evidence of benefits and with case examples of catastrophic outcomes [18]. Part of the parental motivation for consenting to such controversial interventions is to create certainty, when living with uncertainty is often manageable with consistent and quality psychosocial input. Making decisions under duress may be unavoidable in emergencies. In nonemergency situations, health professionals have a responsibility to address the emotional barriers to informed decision making [14]. When a mother with a newborn baby presenting genital differences reflected back to a doctor her emotional struggles in the early days, he said, "We don't need five urologists on our team, we need five psychologists" [19].

Some care providers have likened girls' and women's reaction to the diagnosis of utero-vaginal agenesis (Mayer-Rokitansky-Kuster-Hauser Syndrome, MRKH) as on the spectrum of posttraumatic stress disorder [20]. The incoming information about the body conflicts with internalized gendered expectations. The conflicted and emotive information cannot be coded, matched, stored, and retrieved as usual [21]. In such circumstances, a woman may rush to choose a medical intervention without having processed the relevant information including the non-curative nature of medical interventions. From a psychotherapeutic point of view, a rush into treatment often reflects emotional avoidance, that is, avoidance of the distress of contemplating the diagnosis and its implications.

BOX 5.1

The following comment from a woman with a DSD after her first-time elective vaginoplasty in adulthood suggests insufficient processing of pretreatment information:

"Having to have [ ] having to go to a doctor every year for a physical, rather than [ ] the assumption that, OK, when the surgery's over that's all you get for a lifetime, you know? [ ] And I didn't know that I'd … have to dilate." [22]

Health Professional Factors

Just as emotional distress can impair the patient's/surrogate's understanding of the proposed intervention, clinicians may also be vulnerable to the emotional charge of their interaction with patients or surrogates. Many doctors and nurses in a number of fields find aspects of their work highly stressful. These are often related to the emotive transactions they find themselves in, typically with limited support within their hierarchy or organization. Fuelled by patient distress, the clinician may feel under a great deal of pressure to provide a solution. This may make it more difficult to *decenter* their personal biases, such as those pertaining to normalcy [23]. The care provider may filter in and out certain cues from the patient or misunderstand them, or fail to probe and elicit the patient's subjective appraisal of the condition and treatment options.

The way that the information is presented can have undue influence on the patient's or surrogate's decision making. For example, research shows that a disease narrative of genital differences can lead to more people opting for cosmetic genital surgery, compared to a less medicalized narrative [24]. Health professionals can be unduly optimistic about the impact of their interventions. A study of online advertisements for cosmetic labiaplasty is a case in point [25]. Labiaplasty was presented as an effective treatment for "labial hypertrophy," an unproven construct invented relatively recently. References to vulva appearance diversity, alternative ways for managing body distress and dissatisfaction, and scientific information on benefits and risks were absent from the US and UK provider websites.

Some health professionals may be unduly pessimistic about the patient's ability to manage without treatment. In an attempt to maintain hope, the treating clinician may minimize the risk of physical and/or psychological complications. To avoid putting off patients who have expressed a desire for treatment, the clinician may gloss over the challenging self-managed regime afterward. Furthermore, the ongoing psychological and financial costs of attending medical follow-ups and submitting to clinical procedures can easily be underestimated because, for health professionals who have spent years in clinical environments doing clinical activities, these demands are routine.

Physicians and surgeons trained in an intensive, competitive, and exclusively biomedical subculture may be prone to confuse treatment with care. The idea that many patients are better off untreated may lead to feelings of inadequacy and is resisted. For some clinicians, professional activity may be measured by the amount of treatment done, rather than the quality doctoring that they provide. Payment structures can inadvertently encourage over treatment, when an intervention however equivocal always triggers a cost, whereas expert advice and support for the same patient or family does not. These arrangements can create a situation whereby the only way for a patient or surrogate to access specialist input is to opt into a treatment trajectory [26]. The kind of expert advice and support that is so valuable for patients and families is at risk of being continuously marginalized. These systemic factors may compromise the principles of ethical care, and health professionals so affected would need to challenge the status quo.

Theories of Decision Making

Although decision making is a process, it is not usually sequential. The brain makes decisions by processing the same information simultaneously using systems that have different functions. Mukharjee [27] illustrates the point by differentiating between *System A* and *System D* processing. System A refers to a fast, associative, and affect-based mode of decision making heavily influenced by emotional arousal and mood states. System D is an analytical and logic-based mode of decision making that is typically slower. In general, situations experienced as emotive by the decision maker tend to shift the balance toward System A outputs to gain short-term relief from threat, and away from System D outputs, which may be more advantageous for complex and nuanced decisions.

BOX 5.2

The following advice from a mother of a newborn baby presenting atypical genitalia recommends waiting several months for emotions to return to baseline before making far-reaching treatment decisions for the child:

"Take a few months to recover from childbirth, get your feet back on the ground, and take some time to adapt to the diagnosis. Only then are you in a position to consider properly all the options for your child's care. During that time you learn so much about the diagnosis; it becomes less overpowering and less all-consuming and less frightening." (19)

Treatment providers may erroneously rely on a false assumption that logical deliberations prevail across individuals and clinical scenarios. They may underestimate the influence of affect-based decision making. For a threatening diagnosis such as MRKH for example, the gynecologist is conducting the consultation and presenting information targeting System D, while the patient is receiving and computing the information and expressing a decision in predominantly System A mode. The mismatch ultimately fails to engage the patient or surrogate to deliberate on the full range of possibilities in the immediate and longer term.

Facilitating Informed Decision Making

Psychological theories and research have highlighted some of the barriers to professional practice that transforms ethical principles into ethical behaviors. This section outlines the ways in which certain insights from the behavioral and cognitive sciences can be exploited to enhance clinical practice. A behavioral checklist is provided at the end of this section to ensure consistency of professional behaviors in consenting situations (Table 5.1). A dovetailing guide for patients and surrogates is also provided (Table 5.2).

Information Exchange

Patients and surrogates need to have a good enough understanding of the proposed intervention and the alternatives to weigh their decision. What and how information is shared between the patient and/or surrogate and the clinicians can have a profound influence on the former's ability to make an informed choice. The idea that informed consent is "a process of communication between the physician and patient" [14] is therefore entirely consistent with psychological theories and research. Effective doctor-patient communication is generally considered to be a cornerstone and a "central clinical function" in medicine [28]. Communication skills training is most developed in oncology and for some years mandatory for core members of multidisciplinary cancer services in the UK. Sadly, mandatory communication skills training is rare in other disciplines, reflecting a lack of recognition of the impact that health care interaction may bear on patient welfare and decision making, or a lack of commitment to address this.

Rather than information giving, which connotes a one-way process, it is best to think of the doctor-patient interaction as an information exchange. The terminology explicitly acknowledges the conversation as a fluid exploration of all perspectives. Here, access to complete, accurate, and balanced information including factors that could minimally or significantly impact the immediate and longer-term outcome (e.g., requirement of posttreatment self-management, risk of complications) is foundational. Care is taken to tailor the information to the patient's or surrogate's level of health literacy and language capacity. Information can be presented using a variety of media.

It is crucial to check understanding rather than take it for granted when a patient does not ask questions. In checking understanding, a closed question such as "Do you understand?" will shut down conversation, when a few open questions such as "What seems clear to you so far?" and "What would you like me to expand on?" are more likely to open up discussion.

Suffice it to say that vocabularies about the patient's body or body parts that diminish his or her dignity are to be avoided. The care provider should also anticipate and elicit patient/surrogate concerns. Where treatment is not commonplace, it is especially important for the treatment provider to inform the patient or surrogate about any provider factors that might influence outcome [1]. These provider factors might include specifics about his or her training and experience, that is, how many of the proposed procedures he or she has performed, and whether outcomes vary across treatment centers. If the intervention is conducted in infancy or early childhood, the treating clinician should disclose to the surrogate to what age his or her young patients have been followed up, and what is known and unknown about adult effects including further treatments, lifetime complication rates, and reports of patient dissatisfaction. Patients and families should be informed about peer groups so that they can choose whether and to what extent they wish to engage with others with the same or a similar diagnosis.

Psychological Work-up

As discussed, there is a potential for a mismatch in understanding between care providers and care users [30], which can be compounded by emotional arousal on either or both sides. Under pressure, the typical patient or surrogate may rely on cognitive heuristics such as magnification, minimization, or mental filtering to selectively attend to what has or has not been said. It is important to address any misconceptions so that decisions to accept a proposed intervention are based on tangible benefits for the recipient rather than unrealizable wishes. A mutual understanding of

---

BOX 5.3

The following reflection from a mother of a newborn baby presenting atypical genitalia offers insight into how a well-intentioned team of people can confuse the situation for parents:

"I was exhausted and bewildered. The doctors had lost me at the first hurdle: the introductions. I did not understand their expertise, nor how they were going to 'evaluate' my child, and so I could not begin to understand what was the matter with my child." [19]

BOX 5.4

The following comment from a young woman with cloacal anomalies highlights the importance of checking that the patient understands what is being communicated and encouraged to ask questions:

"I didn't understand all the medical words. Like bladder, bowel, and vagina are ok but urethra, cloacal, and stuff, they don't mean anything and I never used to feel confident to say I didn't understand." [29]

BOX 5.5

The following comment from a young woman with cloacal anomalies reported a reluctance to offer honest feedback because of a strong sense of gratitude to and respect for her treatment providers:

"I look at it like they saved my life really and without them I wouldn't be here. So I don't think I would tell them anything." [29]

expectations would often require a series of guided, open conversations. We refer to this input as a *psychological work-up*, a process whereby a person other than the treating physician conducts a series of conversations involving patient or surrogate and helpful others, allowing the decision to emerge over time without pressure.

Psychological work-ups centralize the individual's actual and projected realities in the immediate and longer term. It is especially relevant if the proposed intervention is elective, high risk, or of uncertain clinical benefits, and perhaps especially important if it involves the challenges of indefinite posttreatment self-management and medical reviews, as well as ongoing financial implications (e.g., regular travels to a center of excellence that is out of area). Here, the clinical team aims to build a professional relationship with the family, perhaps via the same key team member, to learn about the family values and preferences, and any specific struggles – emotional or practical.

If the presumed benefits are primarily psychosocial, it is not possible to realistically assess the likelihood of success without psychosocial expertise. Medical caregivers have a responsibility to identify, refer to, and coordinate psychosocial care for patients and families. However, even when physicians are willing, many institutions in many nations do not provide accessible psychological input.

While psychologists are trained to probe and encourage detailed considerations of all aspects including potential disappointment and regret, a psychological work-up can be carried out by any practitioner with the relevant skills and experience. The key is to involve someone other than the treating clinician and preferably a nonmedical professional. The option of deferring treatment temporarily or indefinitely should be given equal weight in decisional consultations. The patient or family should be encouraged to take notes or to record the information in some other way for discussion with helpful and concerned others. Information on peer support should be provided.

A high-functioning clinical team with members sharing the same goals and values is required for any psychological input to be meaningful and productive. For example, a request for the psychologist to complete an assessment before the date set for treatment is highly suspect. It suggests that the psychological input is in reality anything other than a banal, rubber-stamping exercise. The psychologist has a duty to draw attention to the inappropriateness of such a request and the poor practice that this reflects.

A Behavioral Checklist

Current guidance on the nature and process of obtaining informed consent is based on rich thinking from a number of disciplines. While the principles are clear and understandable, their translation into practice may lack rigor. A behavioral checklist may introduce more consistency to a process that is prone to the erroneous assumption that the giving and receiving of medical and treatment information are essentially neutral, rational, and logical. The process of obtaining informed consent can be described in terms of the discrete behaviors required of each party with the recognition that the behaviors exhibited by one party would influence the expressions of the other, and vice versa [31]. For example, the enthusiastic presentation of an intervention by the treating physician may inhibit further questions from the patient or surrogate and the request for a second opinion. Alternatively, a plea for treatment on the part of the patient is likely to inhibit clear communication of the controversies relating to the intervention. The range of dovetailing behaviors required from both parties for ethical practices is summarized in Tables 5.1 and 5.2.

Conclusion

Medical advances have brought immeasurable health benefits to girls and women. With that, the choices and stresses that face patients and families are unimaginable from times past. In pediatric and adolescent gynecology, girls and women may face lifelong conditions that come with uncertainties and dilemmas, including conflicted decisions relating to medical interventions that are not curative and with unproven long-term physical and mental health benefits. It is

Table 5.1 Professional behaviors to facilitate informed consent to elective interventions

- Consider whether this decision is appropriate for a surrogate, or if it should be made by the patient at a later time
- Provide the patient or surrogate with guidance on informed decision making (see Table 5.2 as an example)
- Find out what the patient or surrogate already knows about the intervention and ask how he or she thinks and feels about it
- Ask what additional information he or she seeks
- Give information about the intervention, a segment at a time, for example:
    - Information about the problem that treatment is targeting
    - Information about the procedure
    - Information about known physical and psychological benefits and risks
    - Information about unknown physical and psychological benefits and risks
    - Information about posttreatment demands including self-management, follow-on investigations, examinations, monitoring, additional procedures
- Check understanding after each information segment; if unsure, ask the patient or surrogate to repeat the information in his or her own words
- Encourage the patient or surrogate to express thoughts and feelings after each information segment, picking up cues that might have meaning for decision making including no treatment or postponement of treatment, especially for a minor
- Discuss the observations with the multidisciplinary team and give due consideration to postponement to enable a child to participate in the decision at a later time; minute the discussion and action points
- Feedback to the patient or surrogate the team discussion
- Create time for the patient to process the implications of the information you have presented
- Offer or encourage second opinion
- Decline a written consent after a single discussion or if there is any doubt about the patient's or surrogate's understanding or freedom to choose

Table 5.2 Guidance for patients and surrogates giving informed consent to elective interventions

- Prepare your questions in advance if at all possible
- Include another family member or close other to help you listen to the information if possible
- Take notes or audio record the information (people typically remember about 30 percent of what doctors say)
- Update the treating clinician about what you know so far and your thoughts and feelings about the information you already have
- Ask direct question
- Listen to the answers
- Tell the clinician what is not clear
- Repeat the information in your own words to check that you have understood what is meant
- Ask the treating clinician about his or her experience in giving the treatment
- If at all possible discuss what is known and not known about the physical and psychological benefits and risks of treatment now and later, and what happens afterward, such as how often will you need to come back to the clinic and for how long, how much will it cost, and what is likely to happen at those clinic visits
- Ask what will you/the child be required to do to manage the impact of the treatment afterward, and what happens if you cannot manage
- Discuss the information with people who are helpful to your situation before making up your mind
- Ask further questions until you are satisfied
- Seek a second opinion for major decisions, or if you are not comfortable with the recommendation
- Decline to sign a written consent after a single discussion
- Decline to sign a written consent if you are not comfortable with the recommendation or any aspect of your interaction with the treatment team
- If you have doubt after signing the consent form and before treatment commences, communicate this clearly with the team

now widely recognized that the ultimate goal of care is not to make people "normal" but to enable them to flourish, so that a whole-person care pathway should be in place before any elective, disputed intervention is even considered.

While the provision of balanced information is pivotal, care providers need to do much more to uphold the principles of informed consent. They need to give themselves time to identify with accuracy and consistency patient/surrogate perceptions, priorities, needs, and expectations to avoid a mismatch in understanding. Dedicated psychological input can support patients and families to cope with intense and conflicting emotions in order to make clear-headed decisions. Such input is most meaningful as part of a comprehensive care program provided by a high-functioning multidisciplinary team able to be transparent about their values and reflect on how they work. In the long run, the ultimate test of professional commitment to ethical practice (as opposed to compliance with mandatory governance procedures) is the integration of an in-depth, high-quality, and ongoing training in bioethics in the core curriculum.

References

1. Tamar-Mattis A, Baratz A, Baratz Dalke K, Karkazis K. Emotionally and cognitively informed consent for clinical care for differences of sex development. *Psychology & Sexuality* (2013). DOI: 10.1080/ 19419899.2013.831215

2. Kahnemen D. *Thinking Fast and Slow*. New York: Farrar, Straus and Giroux, 2011.

3. Judicial Council of California. Civil Jury Instruction 532.

4. Faden R, Beauchamp T, King N. *A History and Theory of Informed Consent*. New York: Oxford University Press, 1986.

5. Hack TF, Degner L, Parker P. The communication goals and needs of cancer patients: a review. *Psycho-Oncology* 2005; **14**: 831–45.

6. Davison SN. Facilitating advance care planning for patients with end-stage renal disease: the patient perspective. *Clinical Journal of the American Society of Nephrology* 2006; **1**(5): 1023–28.

7. Gattellari M, Butow P, Tattersall M. Sharing decisions in cancer care. *Social Science and Medicine* 2001; **52**: 1865–78.

8. Say R, Murtagh M, Thomson R. Patients' preference for involvement in medical decision making: A narrative review. *Patient Education and Counseling* 2006; **60**: 102–14.

9. Butow P, Maclean M, Dunn SM, Tattersall MHN, Boyer MJ. The dynamics of change: cancer patients' preferences for information involvement and support. *Annals of Oncology* 1997; **8**: 857–63.

10. Fine A. Nephrologists should voluntarily divulge survival data to potential dialysis patients: a questionnaire study. *Peritoneal Dialysis International* 2005; **25**(3): 269–73.

11. American Academy of Pediatrics. Informed consent, parental permission, and assent in pediatric practice (RE9510). *Pediatrics* 1995; **95**(2): 314–17.

12. Kon AA. Ethical issues in decision-making for infants with disorders of sex development. *Horm Metab Res* 2015; **47**: 340–43.

13. Tamar-Mattis A. Exceptions to the rule: curing the law's failure to protect intersex infants. *Berkeley Journal of Gender, Law & Justice* 2006; **21**: 59–110.

14. Karkazis K, Tamar-Mattis A, Kon AA. Genital surgery for disorders of sex development: implementing a shared decision-making approach. *Journal of Pediatric Endocrinology and Metabolism* 2010; **23**(8): 789–805.

15. Hester JD. Intersex(es) and informed consent: how physicians' rhetoric constrains choice. *Theoretical Medicine* 2004; **25**: 21–49.

16. Fallowfield L, Jenkins V. Communicating sad, bad, and difficult news in medicine *Lancet* 2004; **363**: 312–19.

17. Paulus MP, Yu AJ. Emotion and decision-making: affect-driven belief systems in anxiety and depression. *Trends in Cognitive Sciences* 2012; **16**(9): 476–83.

18. Davies G, Feder E. (eds). Narrative Symposium: Intersex. *Narrative Inquiry in Bioethics* 2015; **5**(2): 87–150.

19. Magritte E. Working together in placing the long term interests of the child at the heart of the DSD evaluation. *Journal of Pediatric Urology* 2012. http://dx.doi.org/10.1016/j.jpurol.2012.07.011

20. Ehlers A, Clark DM. A cognitive model of post-traumatic stress disorder. *Behaviour Research and Therapy* 2000; **38**: 319–45.

21. Heller-Boersma JG, Edmonds DK, Schmidt UH. Cognitive behavioural model and therapy for utero-vaginal agenesis (Mayer-Rokitansky-Kuster-Hauser Syndrome: MRKH). *Behavioural and Cognitive Psychotherapy*, 2009; **37**: 449–67.

22. Boyle M, Smith S, Liao LM. Adult genital surgery for intersex women: a solution to what problem? *Journal of Health Psychology* 2005; **10**: 573–84.

23. Alderson J, Roen K, Muscarella M. Psychological Care: Addressing the Effects of Sexual and Gender Norms. In SM Creighton, A Balen, L Breech, LM Liao (Eds.), *Pediatric & Adolescent Gynecology: A Problem-Based Approach*. Cambridge University Press, 2017.

24. Streuli JC, Vayena E, Cavicchia-Balmer Y, Huber J. Shaping parents: impact of contrasting professional counseling on parents' decision making for children with disorders of sex development. *J Sex Med* 2013; **10**: 1953–60. DOI:10.1111/jsm.12214.

25. Liao LM, Taghinejadi N, Creighton SM. A content and implications analysis of online advertisements for female genital cosmetic surgery. *BMJ Open* 2012; **2**: e001908. DOI:10.1136/bmjopen-2012-001908.

26. Liao LM, Wood D, Creighton SM. Between a rock and a hard place: parents choosing normalising cosmetic genital surgery for their children. *BMJ* 2015; **351**: h5124.

27. Mukherjee K. A dual system model of preferences under risk. *Psychol Rev* 2010; **177**(1): 243–55.

28. Ha JF, Longnecker N. Doctor-patient communication: a review. *Ochsner Journal* 2010; **10**: 38–43.

29. Liao LM, Baker E, Boyle ME, Woodhouse CRJ, Creighton SM. Experiences of surgical approaches to continence management for cloacal anomalies: a qualitative analysis based on six women. *Journal of Pediatric and Adolescent Gynecology* 2013. DOI: 10.1016/j.jpag.2013.11.011.

30. Platt FW, Keating KN. Differences in physician and patient perceptions of uncomplicated UTI symptom severity: understanding the communication gap. *Int J Clin Prac.* 2007; **61**(2): 303–8.

31. Michie S, van Stralen MM, West R. The behaviour change wheel: A new method for characterising and designing behaviour change interventions. *Implementation Science* 2011; **6**: 42. DOI:10.1186/1748-5908-6-42.

Common Gynecological Symptoms before Puberty in Pediatric and Adolescent Gynecological Practice

Stefanie Cardamone and Sarah M. Creighton

Introduction

Gynecological symptoms are relatively common before puberty, although serious pathology is rare. Nonspecific vulvovaginitis and labial adhesions contribute to a significant proportion of the workload of a pediatric gynecologist. Clinicians must be able to confidently identify and manage these common conditions as symptoms can be prolonged and last for many months before resolution. In addition, clinicians also need to be aware of the rarer causes of vulvar symptoms including dermatological disease, recurrent vulvar ulceration, and genital lesions. Vaginal bleeding is uncommon but can indicate more serious underlying pathology and should be carefully investigated.

Vulvovaginal Symptoms

Vulvovaginal symptoms are the commonest gynecological complaints in a prepubertal child and are the most frequent indication for referral to a pediatric gynecologist. Symptoms may include vulvar pruritus and burning and/or pain and may also be accompanied by complaints of vaginal discharge or in rare cases bleeding. A number of factors predispose the prepubertal girl to vulvovaginal conditions including lack of labial development and fat, absence of pubic hair, an unestrogenized mucosa, a more alkaline vaginal environment, and the close proximity of the vagina to the anus. These factors, often combined with difficulty with hygiene, make the vulvar skin in the prepubertal child particularly sensitive to irritants and infections.

Vulvovaginitis

Vulvovaginitis is the most common cause of symptoms before puberty. The peak age of presentation is between ages 3 and 7. Girls may complain of vulvar pain, pruritus, or dysuria, and parents may notice discharge on the child's undergarments. The discharge may be green or yellow and foul smelling. Typically, examination will reveal a reddened "flush" around the vulva and anus. The skin may be excoriated and discharge may be evident. A culture swab of the perineal area can be taken, although this is often negative or contains nonspecific skin flora or mixed anaerobes from the gut. Most vulvovaginitis is noninfectious (74 percent to 80 percent), and often termed "nonspecific vulvovaginitis." When identified, infectious agents include respiratory pathogens, likely from autoinoculation or enteric pathogens. The most common infective agents identified in prepubertal vaginitis include *group A beta-hemolytic streptococci* and *Hemophilus influenzae*. Others include *Staphylococcus aureus, Moraxella catarrhalis, Streptococcus pneumonia, Niesseria meningitides, Shigella*, and *Yersinia enterolitica* [1]. Specific pathogens should be treated with appropriate antibiotics. Recurrence is common for both nonspecific and infectious vulvovaginitis and the mainstay of treatment is improved vulvar hygiene.

Treatment of Vulvovaginitis

The mainstay of treatment is hygiene and the avoidance of irritants such as soaps. Improvement can be very slow and episodes of recurrent symptoms are common. Parents need to be clear that the measures should be continued long term. It is likely that resolution will occur as the child gets older. This is probably in part due to improved dexterity and skill in keeping the genital area clean. In addition, the rise in estrogen levels as puberty approaches will change the anatomy and skin quality. Parents should be counseled on measures outlined in Table 6.1.

Persistent or Recurrent Symptoms

In the case of persistent or recurrent symptoms despite adequate hygiene measures, particularly if a foul odor or vaginal bleeding is present, a specific infection or the possibility of a vaginal foreign body should be considered (see later). Persistent wetness or

Table 6.1 Treatment of Vulvovaginitis

Measure	Action
Clothing	Wear loose-fitting, cotton underpants
	Avoid tights, leggings, and leotards
Bathing	Allow to sit in warm water for 10–15 minutes daily
	Avoid soap to wash the genital area – no bubble baths!
	Wash hair and body just prior to removing child from tub
	Rinse the genital area well and pat dry
General hygiene	Emphasize wiping front to back
	May sit backward on toilet to avoid pooling of urine within the vagina
	Avoid constipation
Other	Shower after swimming
	Avoid sitting in wet swimsuits for prolonged periods
Emollients	Can use soap-free emollients such as aqueous cream for washing
	Barrier creams may help
	No antifungal creams unless fungal infection confirmed on culture

discharge from an ectopic ureter can be confused with "vaginal" discharge. In the case of upper urinary tract infection, purulent discharge may be present. Most commonly the ectopic ureter empties onto the perineum adjacent to the normal urethra; however, other sites include the cervix, vagina, uterus, and urethra. On examination, a small opening or drop of urine might be visible adjacent to the urethra. Further imaging with renal ultrasound and/or intravenous pyelogram can help with the diagnosis and a referral to a pediatric urologist is indicated.

Other Infective Causes

Infections with sexually transmitted organisms such as *Gonorrhea*, *Chlamydia*, or *Trichomonas*, if detected, indicate sexual abuse. Appropriate referral is necessary and is addressed in detail elsewhere. Vulvar pruritus and pain, particularly with symptoms predominantly at night, can be caused by pinworms (threadworms). If clinically suspected, empiric treatment with a single dose of mebendazole may be helpful. Worms may be visible at the anus or in feces, but the traditional "scotch (sellotape) test" suggested to parents in the past is not usually helpful. Candida vaginitis is a common cause of vulvar pruritus and irritation in estrogenized adolescents and adult women; however, it is uncommon in the toilet-trained prepubertal girl. Misdiagnosis and inappropriate treatment are common. If present on vaginal cultures, candidiasis should prompt consideration of diabetes mellitus in this age group.

Dermatological Causes

Dermatologic conditions, such as atopic dermatitis, psoriasis, and lichen sclerosis may also cause vulvar symptoms. Lichen sclerosus (LS) is a chronic dermatologic condition of unknown etiology. An association exists between LS and autoimmune diseases such as vitiligo, autoimmune thyroid disease, alopecia acreata, and rheumatoid arthritis. LS is often seen in adult women, but 10 percent to 15 percent of cases are seen in children [2]. A hormonal association is suggested due to peaks in the prepubertal and postmenopausal years. Additionally, many girls see an improvement in symptoms with the onset of puberty. Clinically, pruritus is the most common complaint, at times associated with pain, dysuria, or bleeding from erosions or fissures. With rectal involvement, constipation or pain with defecation may be present. The diagnosis is made on examination. LS typically appears as a sharply demarcated, hypopigmented lesion surrounding the vulva and anus. The skin appears thin and atrophic, often described as having a "parchment-paper" appearance. Purpura, fissuring, and erosions may be present. With time, significant scarring including fusion and resorption of the labia minora, introital narrowing, and clitoral phimosis may occur (Figure 6.1). In the prepubertal girl with a typical history and physical examination consistent with LS, biopsy is not necessary. Vulvar biopsy should be reserved for cases when the diagnosis is in question or those not responsive to standard treatment.

Treatment involves potent topical steroid such as 0.05 percent clobetasol propionate. Short courses of high-potency topical steroids appear to be safe, effective, and well tolerated [3]. However, prolonged use can be associated with atrophic skin changes, telangiectasias, secondary infection, and adrenal suppression.

A number of regimens have been suggested and have been shown in case series to lead to good response. No robust data in the pediatric population suggests an ideal treatment regimen. Following disease improvement with an initial twice daily or daily regimen of high-potency steroid, a taper to a lower-potency steroid such as 0.1 percent triamcinolone acetonide then 1 percent hydrocortisone should be considered [4].

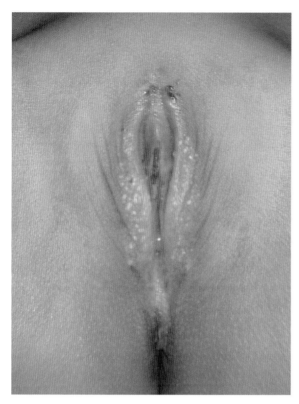

Figure 6.1 Lichen sclerosus

Topical calcineurin inhibitors pimecrolimus and tacrolimus have also been used for treatment of LS. Data regarding their use in this setting is limited; however, multiple case reports have indicated success. A double-blind, randomized prospective study comparing topical clobetasol propionate 0.05 percent with topical tacrolimus 0.1 percent in 55 women and children with LS showed a significant decrease in symptoms (burning, pain, and pruritus) in both groups. However, the clobetasol group showed a significantly faster response in symptom control at one- and two-month follow-up. Moreover, significantly more patients treated with clobetasol achieved complete remission of clinical signs of disease on anogenital exam [5].

Both pimecrolimus and tacrolimus have an FDA black box warning concerning a possible relationship between long-term use and skin cancer and lymphoma. Given the black box warning and the known effectiveness of high-potency steroids for disease management, these should be considered second-line options in the setting of an inadequate response to high-potency steroid following confirmation of a diagnosis of LS with vulvar biopsy. Neither should be utilized in children under age 2.

Even with adequate clinical improvement, recurrence is common and patients should be monitored every 6–12 months to assess for this [6]. Postmenopausal women with lichen sclerosis are known to have an increased risk of squamous cell carcinoma of the vulva. It is uncertain what this risk may be in children and adolescents diagnosed with lichen sclerosis. Parents should be advised of this potential risk and the importance of long-term follow-up for surveillance of symptoms and clinical findings.

Genital Lesions

Prepubertal girls may present with a variety of genital lesions. These may be an incidental finding on routine examination or present as a genital swelling or mass, or at times with pain, irritation, discharge, or bleeding.

Labial Adhesions

Labial adhesions, also known as labial fusion or agglutination, are a common finding in prepubertal girls. The prevalence is likely to be underreported but is cited as between 2 percent and 39 percent [7]. Labial adhesions are uncommon before age 1 and are not present at birth. The etiology is unknown but thought to be due to a combination of vulvar irritation and hypoestrogenism in prepubertal girls. The appearance is characteristic and the diagnosis is made on clinical examination. Fusion of the labial skin is noted extending from the posterior vaginal introitus toward the urethra. There is often a clearly visible raphe consisting of a thin membranous line in the midline where the labia join. In severe fusion, only a pinhole opening may be visible (Figure 6.2). The majority of cases are asymptomatic and no treatment is required. It is thought that 80 percent of cases spontaneously resolve within one year and virtually all will resolve with the onset of puberty and endogenous estrogen production [8]. If symptoms are present, they are often urinary, including frequency, post-void dribbling, and urinary tract infection. There have been rare reports of urinary obstruction. Pooling of urine behind the adhesions may also lead to vulvar irritation and vaginitis.

Treatment of Labial Adhesions

Treatment is only required if the child is symptomatic. First-line therapy should be a conservative approach with topical estrogen. A pea-sized amount of estrogen cream is applied to the labia using a finger or Q-tip with

55

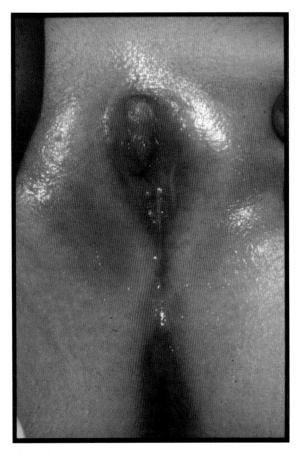

Figure 6.2 Labial adhesions

gentle downward pressure along the line of fusion. The labia will start to "buttonhole" and then separate. Success rates are reported at 50 percent to 88 percent [9]. Once separated, parents should be counseled on vulval hygiene and use of bland emollients to prevent recurrence. However, even with meticulous care, recurrence following discontinuation of treatment is common. Published treatment regimens vary in their frequency and duration of use of estrogen; however, the majority will resolve in 2–6 weeks. Treatment should not exceed 6 weeks as even with topical vaginal administration alone, a small amount of estrogen is absorbed systemically. Although rare, side effects can include breast swelling and tenderness, vulvar pigmentation, and vaginal bleeding. Breast bud formation and vaginal bleeding will resolve after the cessation of treatment.

The use of topical steroid (betamethasone 0.05 percent) has been reported as an alternative or adjuvant conservative therapy for labial adhesions with varying rates of success (16 percent to 89 percent) [10,11].

Betamethasone 0.05 percent can be applied twice daily for 4–6 weeks. Skin atrophy and systemic steroid effects can occur with prolonged use and this should be avoided. Topical estrogen remains the first-line treatment; however, a trial of topical betamethasone can be considered in those who fail estrogen therapy before resorting to surgical separation.

Rarely, in the setting of severe urinary symptoms (urinary obstruction or recurrent urinary infections) and failed conservative management, surgical separation is required. This should be performed under a brief general anesthetic. Manual separation using local anesthesia in the outpatient setting has been reported with good success rates [12]; however, it has been associated with significant distress and discomfort for child and parent alike [13]. If surgical separation is performed, estrogen cream and emollients should be used for a period postoperatively to prevent recurrence. Despite this, recurrence remains common, even after surgery.

Labial Swelling

Less commonly, prepubertal girls may present with swelling or a mass of the genitalia. Initial evaluation should include careful examination noting evidence of a hernia or disorder of sex development. Imaging with ultrasound and, in some cases, MRI can be used for further characterization if indicated. A number of conditions must be considered and can be loosely grouped into conditions that present with focal lesions and those that tend to be less well defined.

Focal Lesions

Focal lesions include hernia, benign tumors such as a polyp, lipoma, neurofibroma, or fibroma, embryonic duct remnants, lymphatic or vascular malformations, hemangioma, and rare malignant tumors such as rhambomyosarcoma. Vaginal or hymenal polyps are rare and may present with bleeding or discharge. Hymenal "skin tags" can be confused with a polyp and are benign. These are often asymptomatic and resolve in time without requiring surgical removal. Hymenal tags can be removed surgically if causing concern such as bleeding or pain, for example, due to tugging with wiping or if increasing in size. Lipomas often present with asymmetry of the labia majora. A discrete mass can be appreciated on gentle palpation and imaging. Treatment is with observation or excision. Vascular malformations are present at birth but may not become clinically evident until later in childhood. Examination may reveal a compressible lesion, often with a bluish discoloration. Pain and thrombosis may be present. Consultation with a vascular surgeon is necessary.

Less Focal Lesions

Less well-demarcated lesions include labial hypertrophy, vulvar edema, and inflammatory etiologies, such as Crohn's disease of the vulva. Childhood asymmetric labium majus enlargement (CALME) is an increasingly recognized entity of unknown etiology that presents with a non-focal enlargement of the labia majora. The etiology is unknown, although neoplastic and an exaggerated hormonal response with pubertal onset have been suggested. Patients will generally present with unilateral swelling of the labia majora with extension centrally to the mons, although bilateral involvement has been reported. On examination there is painless labial swelling without induration or overlying skin changes. When palpated, there is a fleshy consistency without a definable solid or cystic mass. Ultrasound or MRI will reveal ill-defined soft tissue expansion without focal lesion [14]. Although the lesion has historically been resected, the current preferred treatment approach is conservative with clinical and sonographic follow-up [15]. Biopsy and/or excision should be reserved for atypical cases in which the diagnosis is in doubt. Reports of spontaneous resolution have been described and recurrence after resection is common [16].

Vulvar Ulceration

The differential diagnosis of vulvar ulcers is extensive and includes infectious, inflammatory, and rarely malignant etiologies. A thorough history and examination are crucial. Sexual history and concern for abuse should be explored. Clinical features should be detailed including pain, recurrence, medications, and presence of concomitant lesions. Presence of associated symptoms such as fever and malaise may suggest a viral etiology, while gastrointestinal symptoms may suggest a diagnosis of Crohn's disease.

Lipschutz Ulcers

There have been increasing reports of the relatively common occurrence of nonsexually transmitted acute genital ulcers also sometimes called "virginal," aphthous, or Lipschutz ulcers [17]. Lesions generally involve the vaginal introitus and medial labia minora and may be unilateral or bilateral. The ulcers are acutely painful, often >1 cm and appear with raised edges and a denuded, purulent base. In most cases, the ulceration is predated by prodromal viral symptoms that may include fever, malaise, headache, fatigue and/or diarrhea. Viral illnesses such as Epstein Bar virus (EBV), influenza A, and cytomegalovirus (CMV) have been associated with these lesions [18,19]. In many cases a specific etiology is not found; however, investigation for commonly associated illnesses should be performed. A CBC, differential, and serology for EBV should be done. Viral culture and serology for herpes simplex virus (HSV) should be considered although the majority of these cases occur in girls before sexual activity has begun. Depending on the clinical setting, testing for Group A strep and/or influenza may be indicated. Biopsy results are nonspecific and biopsy is not generally needed. Edema of labia minora can be prominent and in some cases can lead to urinary retention. Concomitant oral lesions may also be present consistent with complex aphthosis.

Most girls can be treated at home. Treatment is supportive and includes oral nonsteroidal anti-inflammatory drugs, topical analgesia with lidocaine gel, and Sitz (salt) baths. Patients should be monitored for urinary retention and in some cases placement of a Foley catheter is necessary for urinary drainage. Rarely is admission for pain management necessary. Ulcers often heal within 7–21 days, but recurrence is common. Short courses of tapered oral corticosteroids have been used successfully to shorten duration of symptoms, but clinical studies are lacking.

Herpes Simplex

The lesions of herpes simplex (HSV) should be recognized. In young girls, confirmation of HSV should raise the suspicion of sexual abuse. Patients present with multiple painful vesicular or ulcerated lesions. In a first episode, many patients will have systemic symptoms including fever, malaise, myalgias, and tender inguinal lymphadenopathy. The majority of genital lesions are caused by HSV-2; however, infection from HSV-1 can occur. Type-specific isolation by viral culture is the most accurate means of diagnosis. Treatment is directed toward relief of symptoms with analgesia and oral antiviral regimens. In severe cases, intravenous therapy may be required.

Recurrent Vulvar Ulceration

In the setting of recurrent vulvar ulcers, particularly with oral ulcers or evidence of systemic involvement, the diagnosis of Behcet disease should be considered. Behcet's syndrome is a chronic vasculitis of unknown etiology. The clinical diagnosis requires the presence of oral aphthous ulcers recurring at least three times per year, plus at least two of the following: recurrent genital ulcers, uveitis or retinal vasculitis, skin involvement such as erythema nodosum, or a positive pathergy test.

Fixed drug eruptions can also present with recurrent genital ulcers. These ulcers will occur in the same location each time the offending drug is ingested. Culprits may include NSAIDs, acetaminophen, sulfonamides, tetracycline, phenytoin, or barbiturates. Crohn's disease may have vulvar manifestations including vulvar edema, ulcers, fissures, and/or fistulas. In some cases, vulvar ulcers may precede gastrointestinal symptoms.

Vaginal Bleeding

The differential diagnosis of prepubertal vaginal bleeding is extensive and deserves careful investigation in all cases (Figure 6.3). A careful history and physical examination should focus on duration of bleeding, history of trauma, concerns regarding sexual abuse, signs of pubertal development, history of abnormal bleeding or easy bruising, history of foreign body, and associated vulvar and urinary symptoms. Physical examination involves a general assessment including evidence of height acceleration and pubertal development as well as gynecologic exam taking note of any evidence of vulvovaginitis, trauma, or genital lesions.

The diagnostic evaluation should be guided by the child's clinical presentation. If a diagnosis cannot be reached based on a careful physical examination, vaginal culture should be performed. If vaginal bleeding remains unexplained, examination under anesthesia with vaginoscopy is needed.

In the first week of life, vaginal bleeding can occur due to withdrawal of maternal estrogen. In the older child, causes include vulvovaginitis, vaginal foreign body, urethral prolapse, accidental trauma or sexual abuse, benign and malignant lesions of the genital tract, hemangioma, lichen planus, bleeding disorders, and endocrine causes including precious puberty, precious menarche, and hypothyroidism.

Nonspecific vulvovaginitis rarely causes vaginal bleeding; vaginitis caused by group A beta-hemolytic streptococci (*streptococcus pyogenes*) or Shigella can present with vaginal bleeding. Perineal group A streptococcal infection is classically accompanied by a beefy red, well-demarcated appearance of the infected skin. Vaginitis caused by these organisms requires treatment with appropriate oral antibiotics.

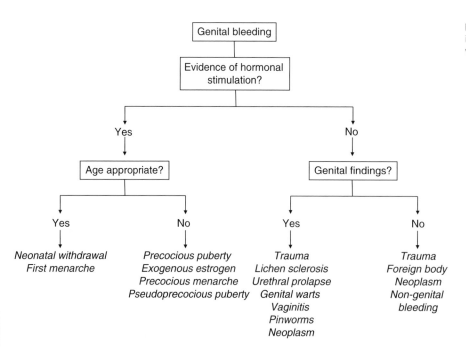

Figure 6.3 Algorithm for the investigation of prepubertal vaginal bleeding

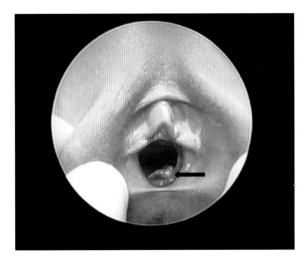

Figure 6.4 Vaginal foreign body

Vaginal Foreign Body

The presence of bleeding, or blood stained discharge, in the absence of a history of trauma, should raise suspicion of a vaginal foreign body [20] (Figure 6.4). Vulvar erythema may be present secondary to chronic discharge. Small fragments of toilet paper are often the culprit, but the cause may include any small objects including beads, small toys, crayon tips, pins, or paper clips. If a small foreign body is visible within the vagina or highly suspected, an attempt can be made to remove the object in an outpatient setting in a cooperative child. Gentle irrigation of the vagina with saline can be performed using a small urethral catheter or pediatric feeding tube attached to a 25 mL syringe. If the patient is not cooperative or the foreign body is not successfully removed, vaginoscopy under general anesthesia is indicated. There is an association between sexual abuse and vaginal foreign bodies, and clinicians need to be alert to this possibility. A history should be taken of possible sexual abuse and swabs taken for sexually transmitted infections at the time of removal of the foreign body.

Urethral Prolapse

Urethral prolapse commonly presents with genital bleeding that may initially be mistaken for vaginal bleeding. Children may also complain of dysuria or pain. Examination will reveal a characteristic annular (doughnut-like), red mass (Figure 6.5). The exact cause of urethral prolapse is unknown, but it is commoner before puberty than after and so may be linked to low levels of estrogen. It is more common in Afro-

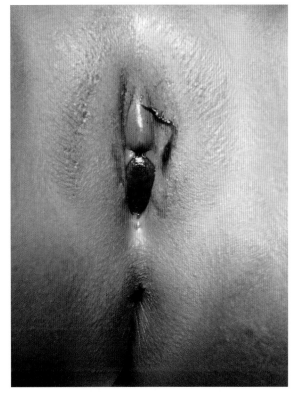

Figure 6.5 Urethral prolapse

Caribbean girls and may be more common in children who have a history of persistent or chronic coughing and constipation [21]. Treating these precipitants is paramount. Urethral prolapse can be treated conservatively as a first line with topical estrogen cream and analgesia [22]. Sitz baths may be helpful. When successful, the prolapse will usually resolve within one to four weeks. When the prolapse persists and is symptomatic, surgical excision is needed.

Genital Trauma

Accidental and abuse-related genital trauma may cause vaginal bleeding. Straddle injuries most commonly result from a fall onto objects such as bicycle frames, furniture, or playground equipment. Bruises, hematomas, and lacerations of the vulva, clitoral folds, labia minora, or periurethral tissue may result. In the case of non-penetrating straddle injuries, the hymen and vagina are usually not involved. Penetrating injuries involving the hymen and vagina can occur if a child falls on a pointed object such as fence posts, furniture, or bath toys or soap dispensers

59

during bath time. Significant vaginal tears can also occur if the vagina becomes over distended with water such as during a water skiing fall or the use of water slides. In the case of over distention injuries, external trauma may be minimal, which can be misleading. An examination under anesthesia is necessary to both identify the source of bleeding and assess the extent of injury. Penetrating injuries in the absence of an appropriate history strongly suggest sexual abuse and the clinician must remain astute.

Superficial lacerations that are not actively bleeding can heal without repair. Otherwise, lacerations should be repaired with the goal of restoring anatomy and achieving hemostasis. Vaginal lacerations in a prepubertal girl can be difficult to suture. In such cases, vaginal packing may be sufficient to stop the bleeding. Small, non-expanding hematomas should be managed with ice, pain relief, and reduced activity. Surgical treatment should be avoided to prevent the risk of infection.

In cases of very large or rapidly expanding hematomas, surgical evacuation is generally required. Evacuation can decrease pain, speed recovery, and decrease the risk of necrosis. The hematoma should be incised on the medial surface near the vagina, the bed debrided, and hemostasis obtained. A small drain should be placed to allow drainage and reduce the risk of infection [23].

If the hematoma is large, the perineal anatomy is significantly distorted, or the child cannot adequately empty her bladder, a Foley catheter should be placed to prevent urinary retention. Bladder drainage should be continued until the swelling resolves. The swelling and discoloration may take several weeks to completely resolve. Large hematomas may result in the tracking of blood along fascial planes along the vaginal wall, pubic symphysis, and lower abdomen.

Benign and Malignant Genital Lesions

Benign and malignant genital lesions may also cause bleeding. Benign lesions such as hemangiomas or urethral or hymenal polyps are easily identified. Condyloma accuminata may bleed and can be congenitally acquired or result from sexual abuse. Although extremely rare, malignancy of the genital tract must always be considered in children presenting with vaginal bleeding. Botyroid sarcoma, or embryonal rhabdomyosarcoma, is a malignant tumor involving the vagina, uterus, bladder, and urethra. The peak incidence is in the first 2 years of life

with 90 percent occurring before age 5. On examination the tumor classically appears as a "grape-like" mass protruding from the vagina or urethra and if identified the child should be referred to the pediatric oncology team.

Conclusions

The majority of prepubertal girls presenting to a pediatric gynecologist will have either vulvovaginitis or labial adhesions. Clinical management involves gentle and thorough assessment and reassurance that no significant pathology is present. Treatment is hygiene based and reassurance of the parents is crucial. Symptoms can be chronic and parents may have seen numerous specialists in the process of seeking a diagnosis. The possibility of child sexual abuse must be considered in cases of chronic symptoms and insertion of a foreign body into the vagina. Clinicians must always remain vigilant. While most gynecological symptoms are easily diagnosed and managed, there are rare causes of significant vulvar pathology such as dermatological disease or rare tumors. In addition, some conditions will require liaison with other specialists, for example, pediatric urology in the case of a suspected ectopic ureter.

References

1. Jacquiery A, Stylianopoulos A, Hogg G et al. Vulvovaginitis: clinical features, etiology, and microbiology of the genital tract. *Arch Dis Child* 1999; **81**: 64–67.

2. Van Eyk N, Allen L, Giesbrecht E et al. Pediatric vulvovaginal disorders: a diagnostic approach and review of the literature. *J Obstet Gynaecol Can* 2009; **31**(9): 850–62.

3. Smith YR, Quint EH. Clobetasol propionate in the treatment of premenarchal vulvar lichen sclerosus. *Obstet Gynecol* 2001; **98**: 588–91.

4. Bercaw-Pratt JL, Boardman LA, Simms-Cendan JS. Clinical recommendation: pediatric lichen sclerosus. *J Pediatr Adolesc Gynecol* 2014; **27**(2): 111–16.

5. Funaro D, Lovett A, Leroux N et al. A double-blind, randomized prospective study evaluating topical clobetasol propionate 0.05% versus topical tacrolimus 0.1% in patients with vulvar lichen sclerosus. *J Am Acad Dermatol* 2014; **71**: 84–91.

6. Focseneanu MA, Gupta M, Squires KC, et al. The course of lichen sclerosus diagnosed prior to puberty. *J Pediatr Adolesc Gynecol* 2013; **26**: 153.

7. McCann J, Wells R, Simon M et al. Genital findings in prepubertal girls selected for nonabuse: a descriptive study. *Pediatrics* 1990; **86**(3): 428–39.

8. Pokorny SF. Prepubertal vulvovaginopathies. *Obstet Gynecol Clin North America* 1992; **19**: 39.

9. Leung AK, Robson WL, Kao CP et al. Treatment of labial fusion with topical estrogen therapy. *Clin Pediatr (Phila)* 2005; **44**(3): 245–47.

10. Eroglu E, Yip M, Oktar T et al. How should we treat prepubertal labial adhesions? Retrospective comparison of topical treatments: estrogen only, betamethasone only, and combination estrogen and betamethasone. *J Pediatr Adolesc Gynecol.* 2011; **24**(6): 389–91.

11. Erturk N. Comparison of estrogen and betamethasone in the topical treatment of labial adhesions in prepubertal girls. *Turk J Med Sci.* 2014; **44**(6): 1103–7.

12. Muram D. Treatment of prepubertal girls with labial adhesions. *J Pediatr Adolesc Gynecol* 1999; **12**(2): 67–70.

13. Smith C, Smith DP. Office pediatric urologic procedures from a parental perspective. *Urology* 2000; **55**(2): 272–76.

14. Gokli A, Neuman J, Lukse R et al. Childhood asymmetrical labium majus enlargement sonographic and MR imaging appearances. *Pediatr Radiol* 2016. [E pub ahead of print] DOI: 10.1007/s00247-016-3543-9.

15. Soyer T, Hancerliogullari O, Pelin Cil A. Childhood asymmetric labium majus enlargement: is a conservative approach available? *J Pediatr Adolesc Gynecol* 2009; **22**: e9–e11.

16. Vargas SO, Kozakewich HP, Boyd TK et al. Childhood asymmetric labium majus enlargement: mimicking a neoplasm. *Am J Surg Pathol* 2005; **29**: 1007–16.

17. Farhi D, Wendling J, Molinari E et al. Non-sexually related acute genital ulcers in 13 pubertal girls: a clinical and microbiological study. *Arch Dermatol* 2009; **145**(1): 38.

18. Huppert JS, Gerber MA, Deitch HR et al. Vulvar ulcers in young females: a manifestation of apthosis. *J Pediatr Adolesc Gynecol* 2006; **19**(3): 195.

19. Wetter DA, Bruce AJ, MacLaughlin KL et al. Ulcus vulvae acutum in a 13-year-old girl after influenza A infection. *Skin Med* 2008; **7**(2): 95.

20. Smith Y, Berman D, Quint E. Premenarchal vaginal discharge: findings of procedures to rule out foreign bodies. *J Pediatr Adolesc Gynecol* 2002; **15**(4): 227–30.

21. Valerie E, Gilchrist BF, Frischer J et al. Diagnosis and treatment of urethral prolapse in children. *Urology* 1999; **54**: 1082–84.

22. Carlson NJ, Mercer LJ, Hajj SN. Urethral prolapse in the premenarcheal female. *Int J Gynaecol Obstet* 1987; **25**: 69–71.

23. Merritt DF. Genital Trauma. In: Emans SJ, Laufer MR. *Pediatric & Adolescent Gynecology*, 6th ed. Philadelphia: Lippincott Williams & Wilkins, 2012.

Chapter 7

Menstrual Dysfunction in Pediatric and Adolescent Gynecology Practice
Heavy Menstrual Bleeding

Michal Yaron and Diane F. Merritt

Introduction

Abnormal uterine bleeding (AUB) and its subgroup heavy menstrual bleeding (HMB) affect 12 percent to 25 percent of reproductive-age women [1,2]. Additionally, HMB affects about 30 percent of adolescent females presenting to the gynecologist [3] and between 10 percent and 100 percent of those with bleeding disorders, depending on the type and severity of the underlying condition [4].

HMB is defined as excessive menstrual blood loss that interferes with the individual's physical, emotional, social, and material quality of life and can occur alone or in combination with other symptoms [5]. A 2006 study showed that HMB affected adolescents' ability to participate in physical education or sports, resulted in at least one day of missed school during each menses, disrupted their hobbies and leisure activities, and increased their level of fatigue [6]. Management of HMB in adolescents must take into consideration the desire to maintain future fertility, contraceptive needs, and improved quality of life.

Definitions

In 2011, the International Federation of Gynecology and Obstetrics published a classification system to describe the causes of AUB in reproductive-age women. This system, which was later adopted by different national societies of obstetricians and gynecologists [7,8], includes the following: acute AUB describes "an episode of heavy bleeding that, in the opinion of the clinician, is of sufficient quantity to require immediate intervention to prevent further blood loss" [9]. Chronic AUB is uterine bleeding that has been present for the majority of the past 6 months. A patient's perception of increased menstrual bleeding may be considered sufficient to make the diagnosis of HMB [9]. In fact, both the Royal College of Obstetricians and Gynaecologists and the

American College of Obstetricians and Gynecologists prefer the patient-centered definition of HMB as an indication for investigation and treatment options. Hence, surrogate objective measurements of volume such as pictorial blood-loss assessment chart scores are not recommended in routine clinical practice [10].

Bleeding is then further categorized according to etiology by using the acronym PALM-COEIN: **P**olyp (AUB-P), **A**denomyosis (AUB-A), **L**eiomyoma (AUB-L), **M**alignancy and hyperplasia (AUB-M) and **C**oagulopathy (AUB-C), **O**vulatory dysfunction (AUB-O), **E**ndometrial (AUB-E), **I**atrogenic (AUB-I), and **N**ot yet classified (AUB-N) [9]. The differential diagnosis of AUB etiology in adolescents is similar to that in adult women; however, proportions of causes differ between the two groups.

Pathophysiology and Differential Diagnosis

The most common cause of AUB in adolescents is ovulatory dysfunction. For the first several years after menarche, some adolescents experience irregular menses due to an immature hypothalamic-pituitary-ovarian axis and subsequent anovulatory cycles [11]. In such cases, the ovaries produce estrogen continuously, hindering ovulation. Without ovulation, no corpus luteum secretes progesterone to stabilize the endometrium. Instead, the endometrium is maintained in the proliferative phase, resulting in thickening and incomplete shedding, which causes irregular, often heavy, menses.

The age at presentation is important when considering etiologies other than an immature hypothalamic-pituitary-ovarian axis. Oligomenorrhea more than 2 years post-menarche is often predictive of persistent cycle irregularity and warrants further assessment to exclude endocrinopathies such as hyperandrogenism, hyperprolactinemia, or thyroid dysfunction. Anovulation may also be induced by obesity.

Severe acute bleeding and heavy menstrual bleeding at menarche with chronic heavy bleeding during the entire reproductive life are common manifestations of inherited or acquired hemorrhagic disorders. In up to 48 percent of cases, adolescents presenting with HMB at or close to menarche (particularly those who require frequent visits to the emergency department, hospital admission, or blood transfusion) have a bleeding disorder, most commonly Von Willebrand disease (vWD) [12,13] (Figure 7A.1). Other medical conditions that can disrupt normal blood clotting and result in HMB include idiopathic thrombocytopenic purpura, hepatitis, chronic renal disease, diabetes mellitus, hypothyroidism, and systemic lupus erythematosus [14].

The presence of regular cycles with moliminal symptoms, such as breast discomfort, cramps, and bloating prior to each menses, are suggestive of ovulatory cycles. Intermenstrual bleeding may suggest an anatomic problem (a partially obstructed outflow tract, for example).

In sexually active adolescents, two common causes of AUB that are not included in the PALM-COIEN classification system are pregnancy-related bleeding (miscarriage, extra-uterine pregnancy) and sexually transmitted infection (STI). STI may lead to cervicitis, endometritis, and pelvic inflammatory disease, resulting in intermenstrual bleeding. Unscheduled endometrial bleeding that occurs during the use of gonadal steroid therapy, "break-through bleeding," is the major component of the AUB-I classification. Iatrogenic causes in adolescents are often related to

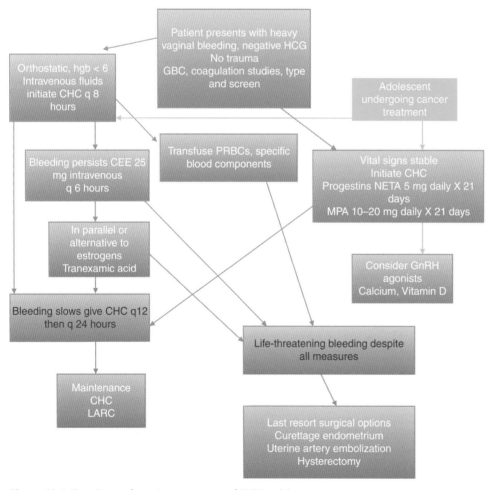

Figure 7A.1 Flow diagram for acute management of HMB in adolescents

contraceptive use, especially long-acting progestin-only methods, or suboptimal compliance with combined oestro-progestatives. Compliance issues include forgetfulness, irregular intake, or concomitant use of medication that reduces contraceptive efficiency [9].

Other mechanisms may cause HMB by disrupting vasculogenesis within the endometrium. These include increased endometrial endothelial cell proliferation, reduced proliferation and differentiation of vascular smooth muscle cells around spiral arterioles, altered synthesis of uterine vasodilatory prostanoids, reduced endothelin expression, and increased expression of endometrial-bleeding-associated factor [1]. An increase in total prostaglandin release and disproportional rise in prostaglandin E2 have also been demonstrated in ovulatory HMB [15,16].

Evaluation

Medical and Menstrual History

Differential diagnosis is aided by the patient's medical history, which should cover the nature of the bleeding, related symptoms that might suggest structural or histological abnormality, impact on quality of life, and full personal medical history. The wide range and natural variability of blood loss in menstrual cycles should be discussed and explained to the adolescent. If uncertain, use of a menstrual calendar or smartphone application may be helpful in objectifying the bleeding pattern. Inquiry should be made about the number of pads or tampons, including their absorbency, used over both a 24-hour period and the whole duration of the menses. Inquiries should be made about heavy bleeding from the onset of menarche, presence of clots (size and frequency), and soaking through clothes or leaking, especially overnight; such symptoms may be associated with a bleeding disorder.

After confirming confidentiality, all adolescents should be privately asked about history of sexual activity, including both consensual and coerced sex.

Further evaluation for blood coagulopathy should be considered if there is family history of an underlying bleeding disorder such as postpartum hemorrhage, surgery-related bleeding, bleeding associated with dental work, and any two of the following symptoms: bruising (1–2/month), epistaxis (1–2/month), frequent gum bleeding, or other bleeding symptoms [14].

Physical Examination

Clinical examination in patients with prolonged or heavy bleeding should always begin with vital signs because tachycardia, hypotension, or orthostatic changes may be the only signs of severe anemia in young patients. A cardiac examination may reveal a flow murmur in anemic patients. Weight and body mass index should be noted. The abdomen should be palpated per usual for masses or hepatosplenomegaly, with special attention on assessing the uterine fundus, which can suggest a pregnancy.

The skin should be examined for bruising and petechia, which would suggest an underlying bleeding disorder; signs of androgen excess (acne, hirsutism, or acanthosis nigricans); and conjunctival or nail bed pallor suggestive of anemia. The patient's thyroid gland should be palpated to detect enlargement or nodules.

In a sexually active adolescent, the physical examination should not differ from that applied to an adult woman. Examination per speculum and bimanual examination can confirm whether bleeding is from the vagina or cervix and is related to trauma, inflammation, or infection (such as cervicitis or pelvic inflammatory disease). However, in the nonsexually active adolescent, assessment would generally not include a speculum or bimanual examination but should rely on external assessment of the genitalia, including the clitoris to assess for signs of virilization, urethral prolapse, active bleeding, or trauma, in accordance with the patient's history [2,7,11,14,17].

Laboratory Investigations

The initial laboratory assessment in adolescents does not differ from that recommended for adult women: screening for pregnancy (urine pregnancy test and/or quantitative serum ß-HCG) is paramount, as not all patients disclose their sexual history despite reassurance about confidentiality. A complete blood cell count (CBC) including differential, platelet count, and a reticulocyte count are essential [11,14]. A serum ferritin test may reflect chronic blood loss and direct replacement therapy but does not provide any more information than a CBC in relation to management of HMB [2,5]. Further testing is directed by history, symptoms, and physical examination.

If a bleeding disorder is suspected, the following tests should be conducted: prothrombin time; activated partial thromboplastin time; fibrinogen; platelet aggregation; and a Von Willebrand panel, which includes Von Willebrand factor (vWF) antigen, ristocetin cofactor assay, and factor VIII [2,5,7,8,17]. Note that vWF is lower in patients with blood type O and during the first three days of menses and higher during pregnancy or when using contraceptives with estrogens.

Thyroid testing should only be performed if signs and symptoms of thyroid disease are present. Female hormone testing should not be carried out on women with HMB, except in patients with irregular cycles or amenorrhea before the onset of the heavy bleeding. In these situations, testing should include follicle stimulating hormone; luteinizing hormone; serum estradiol; total and free testosterone; dehydroepiandrosterone; and, possibly, prolactin to screen for polycystic ovarian syndrome, primary ovarian insufficiency, and hyperprolactinemia [11,14].

Given the high prevalence of STIs in sexually active adolescents, nucleic acid amplification tests for Chlamydia trachomatis and Neisseria gonorrhoeae, either in urine or cervical swabs, are highly recommended [7,18].

Investigation for Structural and Histological Abnormalities

Pelvic sonography, both abdominal (suprapubic) and transvaginal (in sexually active adolescents), is recommended as a first-line procedure to rule out the rare structural cause of AUB in adolescents [2,17], especially when HMB is accompanied by pelvic pain or pressure. Sonography may also delineate endometrial thickness, which is useful in selection of the proper hormonal treatment. Imaging should be undertaken if the uterus is palpable abdominally, vaginal examination reveals a pelvic mass of uncertain origin, or when pharmaceutical treatment fails [2]. Doppler ultrasonography provides additional information useful for characterizing endometrial and myometrial abnormalities [17]. Endometrial biopsy, hysteroscopy, saline infusion sonography, or magnetic resonance imaging are rarely used in adolescents in the context of HMB [7].

Treatment

Principles

The management objectives of AUB are to stop bleeding, restore a stable hemodynamic state, and treat and prevent anemia. Identification of the underlying cause can guide both acute treatment and maintenance therapy to establish regular menses and improve the adolescent's quality of life [2,3,6,7,14,]. (See Table 7A.1.)

Satisfaction and continuation of any given treatment will be influenced not only by efficacy but also by the adolescent's goals and tolerance of side effects. The decision to proceed with any medical treatment should be based on a discussion of patient preference, need for contraception, underlying medical conditions or contraindications, presence of dysmenorrhea, and severity of the bleeding [19].

Medical therapy is the preferred first-line treatment for AUB in adolescents. Irregular or prolonged bleeding is most effectively treated with hormonal options that regulate cycles, thus decreasing the likelihood of unscheduled and potentially heavy bleeding episodes, preserving fertility, and often providing contraceptive benefits.

The criteria for hospitalization are hemodynamic instability, HMB in an already anemic patient, or acute active HMB and a hemoglobin of less than 8 mg/dl in a chronically anemic patient [20,21]. Intravenous crystalloids for blood volume are given initially, but other blood products (clotting factor replacements, platelet transfusions, plasma-derived vWF concentrate, or Factor VII concentrate) and anti-fibrinolytics should be used in specific deficiencies and given judiciously after discussion with the pediatric hematologist.

Hormonal Options

Hormonal therapy is considered first line in the management of AUB in adolescents with or without a bleeding disorder and regardless of sexual activity status. Hormonal treatment is also effective for HMB resulting from fibroids or adenomyosis, though these are uncommon in adolescents. The best choice of hormonal treatment in a given patient depends primarily on endometrial thickness at time of presentation. Progestins are much less effective in patients with thin denuded endometrium.

Estrogen

Estrogen improves homeostasis by promoting endometrial vasospasm and regeneration of denuded epithelial lining and by augmenting clotting factors. Estrogen is given in a combined hormonal contraceptive (CHC) with progestins, which suppresses

Table 7A.1 Treatment options for Heavy Menstrual Bleeding in Adolescents

Treatment	Product	Advantages	Disadvantages

NSAID	Naproxen
	   275–500 mg PO q 6-8 h (US)
	   250–500 mg PO × 2–4/day
	Ibuprofen
	   Up to 1200/day
	Mefenamic acid
	   Initial dose 500 mg the 250 mg q 6 hr
		Self-administered
		Also treats primary dysmenorrhea
		May reduce bleeding
			GI upset (take with food or milk)
			Monitor renal and hepatic function

Iron	Oral ferrous sulfate 325 mg (65 mg elemental iron) multiple preparations are available	Correction of iron deficiency anemia and low iron stores Low cost	GI upset and constipation Poorly tolerated with inflammatory bowel disease
	Intravenous multiple preparations are available	For those who do not tolerate side effects of oral therapy	Transient fever, arthralgias, myalgias, flushing, (rare) anaphylactic reactions
Combined hormone contraception (CHC)	Combined oral contraceptive pill 30–35 mcg EE + Progestin 3 or 4 times a day until bleeding stops then taper dose as bleeding improves to once daily for maintenance Transdermal patch weekly for maintenance Vaginal ring every 3 or 4 weeks for maintenance	Self-administered Provides contraception May use in extended cycles Retain fertility when stopped	In higher doses (3 or 4 times a day) for acute HMB can cause nausea
Estrogen only	Conjugated equine estrogen 25 mg Intravenous every 6 hours* until bleeding stops then transition to oral CHC	Rapid action	Nausea

Progestin only	Medroxyprogesterone acetate
	   10 mg/day for maintenance
	   20–40 mg TID* acute HMB
		Self-administered	Does not provide contraception

	Norethindrone acetate
	   5 mg /day (US) for maintenance
	   10–40 mg/day * acute HMB
		Fertility preserving	

	Depo Medroxyprogesterone acetate Intramuscular 150–300 mg q 12 weeks	Provides contraception	Intramuscular dosing may result in hematoma in at risk patients
	Progestin-only pill	Self-administered Fertility preserving when stopped	Breakthrough bleeding
	Progestin releasing vaginal ring	Self-administered	Break through bleeding Not available in US
	Etonogestrel subdermal implant	Not recommended	Inability to predict bleeding patterns
	LNG IUS for maintenance	Provides contraception Remains 5 year Retain fertility when IUS removed Requires skilled placement	Replace every 5 years May take 6 cycles to relieve HMB

Table 7A.1 (cont.)

Treatment	Product	Advantages	Disadvantages
Antifibrinolytics	Tranexamic acid Oral 1 gram X 3–4/day Oral 650 mg two tablets TID (US) Intravenous 10 mg/kg every hours	Non-invasive Self-administered Retain fertility throughout	May increase chance of clot or stroke if combined with CHC Will not induce amenorrhea
Anti-diuretic hormone	Desmopressin acetate 0.3 mcg/kg IV over 15–30 minutes 150–300 mcg intranasal	Use in mild to moderate von Willibrand disease (type I) and Hemophilia A with factor VIII levels >5%	Contraindicated with history hyponatremia Monitor renal function
GnRH agonists	Leuprolide acetate (for cancer patients) Ideally start before induction of myelosuppressive therapy and 4 weeks before the onset of thrombocytopenia Intramuscular 3.75–7.5 mg/month 11.25–22.5 mg IM every 3 months Subcutaneously 3.75 mg		Initial rise in circulating GN and sex steroids (flare) Long term use increases osteoporosis risk Consider add-back with estrogens or calcium and Vitamin D

ovulation and causes the endometrium to atrophy, thus protecting it from unopposed estrogen and consequently hyperplasia or carcinoma.

Nausea, a common side effect of high-dose estrogen, should be mitigated by anti-nausea medications as needed. To date, no data are available to recommend one specific type of CHC over any other [8,11,22].

In an unstable patient who is unable to tolerate oral medications or continues to bleed despite maximal oral therapy, intravenous or intramuscular conjugated equine estrogen may be indicated [7,27]. Thereafter, patients should be transitioned to maintenance therapy with CHC (oral, patch, or ring) via a tapering regimen [13,22,23]. Adolescents with HMB may benefit from extended cycle regimens. CHCs may confer risk of blood clot, so contraindications should be well respected (24).

Progestin Only

For patients with a contraindication to estrogen products, progestin-only contraceptives can effectively treat HMB [25]. While short courses (7–10 days) of luteal phase oral progestins alone are not effective for the treatment of HMB (5), long-cycle (>21 days) oral progestins such as norethindrone acetate (NETA) or medroxyprogesterone acetate (MPA) have been shown to reduce HMB. Progestin-only pills may also be useful, though they have not been thoroughly studied for treatment of AUB [7]. Compared to oral NETA, the progestogen-releasing vaginal ring (not currently available in the United States) did not show significant superiority in reducing blood loss but was more acceptable to patients [24,26]. In the acute setting, high-dose oral MPA, NETA, or depo-MPA intramuscularly combined with 3 days of oral MPA 20 mg every 8 hours for 9 doses may be used [28].

For maintenance therapy, lower doses (10 mg MPA or 5 mg NETA) should be used for at least 3 to 4 weeks [2,7,14,17,27], or depo-MPA 150 mg (intramuscularly or subcutaneously) every 3 months. The subcutaneous form allows for safe and effective administration in patients with blood dyscrasia at risk for developing hematomas at injection sites [6,18]. Treatment with subcutaneous progestins causes amenorrhea in 41 percent to 47 percent of patients at 1 year. Nevertheless, MPA is less efficient than tranexamic acid (described later) [26].

The levonorgestrel intrauterine system (LNG-IUS) is now considered one of the most effective and cost-effective medical treatments for HMB and is safe in adolescents [7,26,29,30,31]. The LNG-IUS exposes the endometrium to continuous progestogen, causing atrophy and up to 80 percent reduction in menstrual bleeding at 6 months and more than 90 percent by 12 months [27]. IUS users should be advised of anticipated changes in the bleeding pattern, particularly in the first few cycles, and should be encouraged to continue for at least six cycles to see the benefits of treatment. The LNG-IUS has been effective in treating HMB among adolescents with bleeding disorders that are refractory to other treatments [6,9,29,30,31] and was shown to significantly improve quality-of-life measures more than other medical therapies (26,28,29). Recent data suggest that continuation rates for LNG-IUS in women younger than age 20 are comparable to rates of older women [32,33].

Danazol and gonadotropin releasing hormone (GnRH) agonists are generally not recommended for adolescents because of their side effects. They could be used in severe HMB or when further endometrial suppression is required for symptomatic relief and to correct anemia before a final treatment decision can be made.

Nonhormonal

Iron Supplements

Adolescents with HMB resulting in anemia or low iron stores should be encouraged to take supplemental iron and eat iron-rich foods [5]. Some recommend folate supplementation and multivitamins in patients with severe anemia [19].

Tranexamic Acid

Women with HMB have elevated endometrial levels of plasminogen activators, which cause degradation of blood clots, or fibrinolysis. Tranexamic acid is an antifibrinolytic agent that reversibly binds to plasminogen to reduce local fibrin degradation without changing blood coagulation parameters [34]. Tranexamic acid is an effective treatment for HMB and improves quality of life in affected women [7,8,25,34].

The dose of tranexamic acid for the treatment of cyclic HMB in the United States is 1,300 mg (two 650 mg tablets) orally three times a day (3,900 mg/day) for a maximum of 5 days during monthly menstruation. In Europe, the standard treatment regimen is 1 g of tranexamic acid taken orally every 6 hours during menstruation, but a single daily dose of 4 g is also effective. Intravenous tranexamic acid is available for more acute scenarios but should be used with caution in patients with impaired renal function or history of thromboembolic disease.

Nonsteroidal Anti-Inflammatory Drugs (NSAIDs)

The endometrium of women with HMB contains increased levels of prostaglandin E2 and prostaglandin F2α. NSAIDs (e.g., naproxen, ibuprofen, and mefenamic acid) inhibit the enzyme cyclooxygenase, thereby reducing prostaglandin levels. A 2013 Cochrane review showed that NSAIDs more effectively treat HMB than placebo but are not as effective as tranexamic acid or LNG-IUS [35]. Therapy ideally begins the day prior to menses and continues for 2–4 days or until bleeding stops. NSAIDs have the added benefit of improving dysmenorrhea. However, adolescents with HMB and a history suspicious for bleeding disorders should be instructed to avoid NSAIDs, aspirin, heparin, and platelet-inhibiting substances until a work-up is completed [22].

Synthetic Analogue of Vasopressin (1-desamino-8-D-arginine Vasopressin, DDAVP)

DDAVP as a nasal spray or intravenously has been shown to improve bleeding symptoms in patients with vWD and prolonged bleeding time with no bleeding disorder. DDAVP alone is highly efficient in patients with type I vWD but is less effective in patients with types II and III. Patients using DDAVP should restrict fluid intake. In patients with severe acute HMB requiring significant fluid replacement, DDAVP should be avoided because of risk of hyponatremia [36].

With exception of NSAIDS the same medical agents used to treat HMB in women with normal coagulation can effectively be used in the setting of inherited bleeding disorders [7].

Unable to Treat Medically or Failure of Medical Treatment

Surgery is rarely necessary in adolescents with HMB as greater than 90 percent will respond to medical management [23]. If bleeding is continuous and life threatening and the patient is unresponsive to 1–2 days of hormonal therapy, dilation and curettage may be necessary, especially when a histopathologic diagnosis is needed [22]. However, case series have demonstrated that dilation and curettage can increase bleeding complications in adolescents with bleeding disorders. Uterine artery embolization and endometrial ablation are reserved for life-threatening cases because they may impair future fertility [22]. Other beneficial procedures with less adverse effects include placement of an intrauterine 26F Foley catheter infused with 30 ml of saline or uterine packing to tamponade the uterus mechanically. Other surgical procedures including hysteroscopy, endometrial ablation, and hysterectomy are extremely rarely used in adolescents and are only indicated when a rare structural anomaly (e.g., polyp or fibroid) requires resection, or loss of fertility is weighed against loss of life by exanguination [19,36,37].

Other Medical Conditions

Many patients seen by pediatric and adolescent gynecologists have special physical, intellectual, or psychological needs that require thoughtful consideration. The menstrual history should be carefully reviewed to determine the impact of HMB on the adolescent's health and well-being. The ability of a young girl to manage her personal hygiene with or without a caregiver's assistance is a necessary concern. Management of HMB and personal hygiene may be especially difficult when a person is immobile, confined to a wheelchair, or has poor hand coordination [38,39].

Often the caregiver requests menstrual management and should be reminded that monthly menses are a sign of health; once regular cycles are established, many young women are able to provide self-care and manage necessary hygiene issues. However, many patients rely entirely on their caregivers for all hygiene issues. If protective garments (diapers) are used, placing a sanitary pad in the diaper is an option. Trimming (not shaving) of the pubic hair will also help with ease of hygiene.

Menstrual Suppression

Many caregivers will request complete menstrual suppression or even hysterectomies for their daughters. As long as there are no contraindications to estrogen such as a hypercoagulable state or migraines with aura, options for medical treatment include extended cycle estrogen-progestin contraception, cyclic estrogen-progestin contraception with estrogen in place of placebo pills, or natural cycles with targeted supplemental estrogens during menses. In one study, targeted use of the 0.1 mg transdermal estradiol/24-hour patch during menses was effective in decreasing menstrual flow, but lower doses of estradiol were not [40]. Continuous use of the intravaginal contraceptive ring may result in amenorrhea. Menstrual suppression can also be attained with progestin-only pills; nevertheless, breakthrough spotting/bleeding may occur even with optimal compliance. Daily oral NETA 5 mg, injections of depot- MPA, and long-acting reversible contraceptive methods should also be considered. If a patient tolerates blood draws, she should tolerate placement of a subcutaneous implant.

Placement of an LNG-IUS may require sedation and, for convenience, may be coordinated with other sedated procedures such as dental care, eye exams, or port placement. Patients who are receiving tube feedings can receive oral medications via that route. Transdermal contraceptive patches or subcutaneous implants can be impractical if a patient scratches or picks uncontrollably.

HMB is almost always managed medically, and use of hysterectomy is an irreversible, sterilizing, costly, and potentially risky procedure. The American College of Obstetricians and Gynecologists "asserts that involuntary sterilization is not ethically acceptable because of violation of privacy, bodily integrity, and reproductive rights" [39]. Likewise, the Ashley treatment, which combines early estradiol exposure to limit growth, a hysterectomy to prevent menses and pregnancy, and preemptive breast removal, has provoked much debate and remains ethically controversial [41].

HMB and Exacerbation of Underlying Medical Conditions with Catamenial Symptoms

Catamenial Seizures and Hormone Use with Antiepileptics

Estrogen production at puberty onset enhances the seizure activity of young women, whereas progestogens decrease the tendency to have seizures. Thus, progestin-only CHCs, oral and injectable MPA, NETA, and the progestin-containing intrauterine devices and implants are favored for young women who need cycle control or contraception.

Catamenial Migraines

Menstrual migraines, which occur within two days before the onset and through the third day of menstrual bleeding are thought to be due to low endogenous levels of estrogen and are treated the same as migraines occurring at other times. Menstrual migraines can be treated with NSAIDs and triptans and can be prevented via estrogen-containing menstrual suppression as described earlier.

Catamenial Behavioral Disorders

Developmentally impaired adolescents may have cyclic behavior changes including aggressive or self-abusive behavior, tantrums, withdrawal, or crying spells. Dysmenorrhea is often the underlying cause, so initial treatment with NSAIDs is reasonable. Data regarding the use of selective serotonin reuptake inhibitors for premenstrual dysphoria and menstruation-associated depression in adolescents are limited, though fluoxetine should be considered the best available choice when a pharmacological treatment is indicated for moderate to severe depression in people younger than age 18 [42]. Hormonal suppression of ovulation as described earlier is also a viable option.

Options for Preventing and Managing HMB in Adolescents Undergoing Cancer Treatment

In an adolescent undergoing cancer treatment, menstrual bleeding can be compounded by myelosuppression from chemotherapy and radiation therapy. Thus, the patient's oncologist and gynecologist should consult before initiation of chemotherapy or during a time of heavy bleeding. Options for menstrual suppression include CHC, progestin-only therapy, and GnRH agonists. However, GnRH agonists should be given only after 5–7 days of CHC; if given alone, they may exacerbate uterine bleeding after the first dose. When GnRH agonists are used, patients should be advised to take calcium and vitamin D supplements. If use is anticipated for longer than 6 months, add-back hormonal therapy is also necessary to mitigate risk of osteopenia. Urgent need to stop HMB may be accomplished with hormonal therapy or antifibrinolytics [43].

The ideal treatment for acute life-threatening bleeding has not been established, but a suggested algorithm is found in Figure 7A.1. Management of HMB in adolescents with and without special medical conditions requires an understanding of the pathophysiology involved, thoughtful consideration of the many options for treatment, and long-term commitment to the need to preserve future fertility and quality of life for adolescents and young women.

References

1. The ESHRE Capri Workshop Group. Endometrial bleeding. *Hum. Reprod. Update* (2007); **13**(5): 421–31.

2. Sokkary N, Dietrich J. Management of heavy menstrual bleeding in adolescents. *Curr Opin Obstet Gynecol* 2012; **24**: 275–80.

3. Benjamins LJ. Practice guideline: evaluation and management of abnormal vaginal bleeding in adolescents. *J Pediatr Health Care.* 2009; **23**(3): 189–93.

4. Dietrich JE, Yee DL. Thrombophilic conditions in the adolescent: the gynecologic impact. *Obstet Gynecol Clin North Am* 2008; 36–163.

5. National Collaborating Centre for Women's and Children's Health. Commissioned by the National Institute for Health and Clinical Excellence. *Heavy Menstrual Bleeding.* London: RCOG Press at the Royal College of Obstetricians and Gynecologists. First published 2007.

6. Wang W, Bourgeois T, Klima J et al. Iron deficiency and fatigue in adolescent females with heavy menstrual bleeding. *Haemophilia.* 2013 Mar; **19**(2): 225–30.

7. Singh S, Best C, Dunn S et al. Clinical Practice – Gynecology Committee et al., Society of Obstetricians and Gynaecologists of Canada. Abnormal uterine bleeding in pre-menopausal women. *J Obstet Gynaecol Can.* 2013; **35**(5): 473–79.

8. The American College of Obstetrics and Gynecologists. Management of acute abnormal uterine bleeding in nonpregnant reproductive-aged women. Committee Opinion Number 557. *Obstet Gynecol* 2013; **121**: 891–96.

9. Munro MG, Critchley HO, Broder MS et al. FIGO classification system (PALM-COEIN) for causes of abnormal uterine bleeding in nongravid women of reproductive age. *Int J Gynaecol Obstet* 2011; **113**: 3–13.

10. Whitaker L, Critchley HOD. Abnormal uterine bleeding. *Best Practice & Research Clinical Obstetrics and Gynecology* (2015), http://dx.doi.org/10.1016/j.bpobgyn.2015.11.012

11. Deligeoroglou E, Karountzos V, Creatsas G. Abnormal uterine bleeding and dysfunctional uterine bleeding in pediatric and adolescent gynecology. *Gynecol Endocrin* 2012; **29**(1): 74–78.

12. James AH, Manco-Johnson MJ, Yawn BP et al. Von Willebrand disease: key points from the 2008 National Heart, Lung, and Blood Institute guidelines. *Obstet Gynecol* 2009; **114**(3): 674–78.

13. Kulp JL, Mwangi CN, Loveless M. Screening for coagulation disorders in adolescents with abnormal uterine bleeding. *J Pediatr Adolesc Gynecol* 2008; **21**(1): 27–30.

14. Bennett AR, Gray SH. What to do when she's bleeding through: the recognition, evaluation, and management of abnormal uterine bleeding in adolescents. *Curr Opin Pediatr.* 2014; **26**(4): 413–19.

15. Milling Smith OP, Jabbour HN, Critchley HOD. Cyclooxygenase enzyme expression and E series prostaglandin receptor signalling are enhanced in heavy menstruation. *Human Reproduction* 2007; **22**(5): 1450–56.

16. Smith SK, Abel MH, Kelly RW et al. Prostaglandin synthesis in the endometrium of women with ovular

dysfunctional uterine bleeding. *Br J Obstet Gynaecol.* 1981; **88**(4): 434–42.

17. Marret H, Fauconnier A, Chabbert-Buffet N et al. CNGOF Collège National des Gynécologues et Obstétriciens Français. Clinical practice guidelines on menorrhagia: management of abnormal uterine bleeding before menopause. *Eur J Obstet Gynecol Reprod Biol.* 2010; **152**(2): 133–37.

18. Management of Acute Abnormal Uterine Bleeding in Nonpregnant Reproductive-Aged Women. Committee Opinion Number 557. The American College of Obstetrics and Gynecologists. *Obstet Gynecol* 2013; **121**: 891–96

19. Ray S, Ray A. Non-surgical interventions for treating heavy menstrual bleeding menorrhagia) in women with bleeding disorders. *Cochrane Database of Systemic Reviews.* 2014, Issue 11. Art. No.: CD010338.

20. Chi C, Pollard D, Tuddenham EG, Kadir RA. Menorrhagia in adolescents with inherited bleeding disorders. *J Pediatr Adolesc Gynecol.* 2010; **23**(4): 215–22.

21. Wilkinson JP, Kadir RA Management of abnormal uterine bleeding in adolescents. *J Pediatr Adolesc Gynecol.* 2010; **23**(6 Suppl): S22–30.

22. James AH. Bleeding disorders in adolescents. *Obstet Gynecol Clin North Am.* 2009; **36**(1): 153–62.

23. American College of Obstetricians and Gynecologists. Menstruation in girls and adolescents: using the menstrual cycle as a vital sign. Committee Opinion Number 651. *Obstet Gynecol* 2015; **126**: e143–46.

24. World Health Organization. *Medical eligibility criteria for contraceptive use*, 5th ed. Geneva, Switzerland: World Health Organization; 2015. http://who.int/repro ductivehealth/publications/family_planning/MEC-5/en/

25. National Institute for Health and Care Excellence. Heavy menstrual bleeding: investigation and treatment. Surveillance proposal guidance executive document. www.nice.org.uk/guidance/cg44/resources/ heavy-menstrual-bleeding-surveillance-review -decision-march-20153. Published January 2007.

26. Lethaby A, Irvine GA, Cameron IT. Cyclical progestogens for heavy menstrual bleeding. *Cochran Database of Systematic Reviews* 2008, Issue 1, Art. No.: CD001016.

27. DeVore GR, Owens O, Kase N. Use of intravenous Premarin in the treatment of dysfunctional uterine bleeding – a double-blind randomized control study. *Obstet Gynecol.* 1982; **59**(3): 285–91.

28. Ammerman SR, Nelson AL. A new progestogenonly medical therapy for outpatient management of acute, abnormal uterine bleeding: a pilot study. *Am J Obstet Gynecol.* 2013; **208**(6): 499; e1–5.

29. Gupta J, Kai J, Middleton L et al. www.ncbi.nlm.nih .gov/pubmed/?term=ECLIPSE%20Trial%20Collabora tive%20Group%5BCorporate%20Author%5D ECLIPSE Trial.

30. Collaborative Group. Levonorgestrel intrauterine system versus medical therapy for menorrhagia. *N Engl J Med.* 2013; **368**(2): 128–37.

31. American College of Obstetricians and Gynecologists. Adolescents and long-acting reversible contraception: implants and intrauterine devices. Committee Opinion Number 539. *Obstet Gynecol* 2012; **120**: 983–88. Reaffirmed 2014.

32. Matteson KA, Rahn DD, Wheeler TL 2nd et al. Society of Gynecologic Surgeons Systematic Review Group. Nonsurgical management of heavy menstrual bleeding: a systematic review. *Obstet Gynecol.* 2013; **121**(3): 632–43.

33. Lethaby A, Hussain M, Rishworth JR et al. Progesterone or progestogen-releasing intrauterine systems for heavy menstrual bleeding. *Cochrane Database of Systematic Reviews* 2015, Issue 4. Art. No.: CD002126.

34. Peipert JF, Zhao Q, Allsworth JE et al. Continuation and satisfaction of reversible contraception. *Obstet Gynecol* 2011; **117**: 1105–13.

35. Bradley LD, Gueye NA. The medical management of abnormal uterine bleeding in reproductive-aged women. *Am J Obstet Gynecol* 2016; 31–44.

36. Lethaby A, Duckitt K, Farquhar C. Non-steroidal anti-inflammatory drugs for heavy menstrual bleeding. *Cochrane Database of Systematic Reviews* 2013, Issue 1. Art. No.: CD000400.

37. Marjoribanks J, Lethaby A, Farquhar C. Surgery versus medical therapy for heavy menstrual bleeding. *Cochrane Database of Systematic Reviews* 2016, Issue 1. Art. No.: CD003855.

38. Aletebi FA1, Vilos GA, Eskandar MA

39. Thermal balloon endometrial ablation to treat menorrhagia in high-risk surgical candidates. *J Am Assoc Gynecol Laparosc.* 1999; **6**(4): 435–39.

40. American College of Obstetricians and Gynecologists. Menstrual manipulation for adolescents with disabilities. ACOG Committee Opinion Number 448. *Obstet Gynecol* 2009; **114**: 1428–31. Reaffirmed 2012.

41. American College of Obstetricians and Gynecologists. *Reproductive Health Care for Adolescents with Disabilities.* Supplement to guidelines for adolescent health care, 2nd ed., 2012.

42. MacGregor EA, Frith A, Ellis J et al. Prevention of menstrual attacks of migraine: a double-blind placebo-controlled crossover study. *Neurology.* 2006; **67**(12): 2159.

43. Kerruish N. Growth attenuation therapy. *Cambridge Quarterly of Healthcare* Ethics (2016); **25**: 70–83. doi:10.1017/S0963180115000304.

44. Shilyansky C, Williams LM, Gyurak A et al. Effect of antidepressant treatment on cognitive impairments associated with depression: a randomised longitudinal study. *Lancet Psychiatry* 2016; **3**: 425–35.

45. American College of Obstetricians and Gynecologists. Options for prevention and management of heavy menstrual bleeding in adolescent patients undergoing cancer treatment. Committee Opinion Number 606. *Obstet Gynecol* 2014; **124**: 397–402.

Menstrual Dysfunction in Pediatric and Adolescent Gynecology Practice

Common Surgical Causes of Pelvic Pain in the Pediatric and Adolescent Gynecology Patient

Anne-Marie Amies Oelschlager, Lina Michala, and Jennifer E. Dietrich

Background

Pelvic and abdominal pain is common in the pediatric and adolescent population. The differential diagnoses are broad and include gynecologic as well as gastro-intestinal, urologic, musculoskeletal, neurologic, and psychiatric causes (Table 7B.1). Dysmenorrhea, in particular, is a common symptom among adolescents, affecting almost 70 percent of girls [1,2]. Primary dysmenorrhea, painful menstruation that cannot be attributed to pelvic pathology, is thought to be caused by an overproduction of uterine prostaglandins (PGs), which lead to increased myometrial contractility during menstruation. All women have increased levels of PGs during the luteal phase, and these rise

further when the corpus luteum regresses at the onset of menstruation [3]. Typical primary dysmenorrhea lasts for up to 3 days during menstruation; radiates to the lower back or the thighs; and can be accompanied by gastrointestinal symptoms, such as diarrhea or vomiting. The gynecologist needs to assess the like-lihood of whether a patient's pain is related to primary dysmenorrhea or a secondary etiology, including a congenital, physiologic, acquired, or inflammatory process, which may require additional investigation and intervention. The purpose of this chapter is to focus on the conditions that will most likely require gynecologic surgical intervention, which include con-genital anomalies, ovarian cysts, and endometriosis.

Table 7B.1 Causes of pelvic pain in pediatric and adolescent females

Causes of pelvic pain	Location	Etiology
Gynecologic	Ovarian and tubal	Physiologic (follicular cyst, hemorrhagic cyst) Tumors (epithelial, germ cell, sex steroid tumors) Inflammatory (pelvic inflammatory disease, tubo-ovarian abscess) Pregnancy (ectopic pregnancy)
	Uterine	Physiologic (primary dysmenorrhea) Congenital (cervical atresia, obstructed uterine horn) Inflammatory (endometritis) Pregnancy (spontaneous abortion, labor)
	Vaginal	Congenital (vaginal septum, distal vaginal atresia, obstructed hemivagina, imperforate hymen) Inflammatory (vaginitis, chemical irritant) Foreign body (retained tampon, IUD expulsion)
	Vulvar	Inflammatory (vestibulitis, vulvitis, chemical irritant) Trauma and sexual assault
Urologic		Interstitial cystitis, urinary tract infection, nephrolithiasis, urethritis
Musculoskeletal/neuropathic		Hernia, spine anomaly, trauma, neuropathy
Gastrointestinal		Appendicitis, constipation, inflammatory bowel disease, irritable bowel syndrome
Psychiatric		Somatization disorder, pain processing disorder

Initial Evaluation

To begin the evaluation, the patient and her caregivers should be included in the discussion and be asked about the onset of pain (acute, onset less than 3 months, more than 3 months). The patient should be asked where the pain is located and, if possible, she should be asked to point directly to the site of the worst pain. A comprehensive review of systems should be included with specific questions about stool consistency, dysuria, hematuria, rectal pain, anorexia, weight loss, vomiting, fever, back pain, or pain radiating down the legs. The patient should be asked about a history of a large gush of blood; urinary frequency, urgency, or retention; or a sense of needing to defecate without being able to do so, all of which may indicate an obstruction. She should also be asked about any interventions that have alleviated the pain, including specific medications, and any factors that have exacerbated the pain (certain foods, activities, or stress).

A detailed pubertal and menstrual history should be obtained, including age of thelarche, pubarche, and menarche. She should be asked about whether her cycles are regular (every 24–45 days in adolescence), abnormal in length (fewer than 3 days or longer than 7 days), or associated with abnormally heavy flow (passing clots larger than 2–3 cm in diameter or soaking through clothing). She should be asked if she has noted any association with her menstrual cycle (mid-cycle pain, premenstrual pain, or menstrual pain). She should be asked about any precocious or delayed pubertal milestones (early thelarche, delayed menarche), prior ovarian cysts, prior pregnancies, or other medical conditions that may be associated with a decreased pain sensitivity threshold (anxiety, depression, or pain-processing disorder).

A careful past medical history should include specific questions about congenital anomalies including renal, spine, cardiac, anorectal, and ear anomalies. Finally, prior to any medical or surgical intervention, she should be asked about medical conditions with relative or absolute contraindications to menstrual suppression options (migraines, hypertension, and prior arterial or venous thrombosis). Information should be sought about current medications, with particular attention paid to medications that may interact with systemic hormonal treatments. If she has tried hormonal methods for menstrual or ovulation suppression previously, she should be asked whether these medications improved her symptoms and about any side effects that she may have experienced. A detailed history of prior operative interventions should be noted, particularly for patients with anorectal malformations or prior ovarian operations. The family history questions should include questions regarding congenital anomalies, endometriosis, ovarian cancer, thrombophilia, and inflammatory bowel disease.

She should be interviewed privately to discuss her social and sexual health. It is critical that this information be asked without the caregivers present to protect patient confidentiality and improve the ability for the patient to speak freely. She should be asked about her home situation, education, disordered eating, drug use, gender identity and sexuality and whether she is involved in consensual sexual activity or has a history of sexual assault. Her history of current and past contraceptive use as well as prior sexually transmitted infection testing and treatment should be detailed. She should be asked directly about any home or school stress, any current anxiety and depression, and how much the symptoms have limited her ability to attend school and participate in her normal activities.

Physical Examination

At this point, a careful physical exam should be performed. The patient's vital signs and general appearance should be assessed for evidence of acute discomfort or hemodynamic instability. A breast and pubic hair examination will determine her sexual maturity rating. The abdominal exam should include superficial and deep palpation to assess for evidence of peritonitis or the presence of a large mass or advanced pregnancy. The pelvic exam can be stressful and painful for a young adolescent and should be explained to the patient, so that she understands the purpose. Often examination of the external genitalia will permit adequate visualization of the vestibular glands and the distal vagina. Using downward traction of the labia minora, the distal vagina can be examined to assess for patency of the hymen or distal vaginal atresia. A cotton swab can be used to palpate the vestibular glands for tenderness and then inserted into the vagina until resistance is met to assess the depth of the vagina. If the patient is sexually active and consents to an internal vaginal speculum exam, a smaller speculum, such as the Huffman, may be less uncomfortable than typical adult size speculums. A digital bimanual examination can be performed to assess for cervical motion tenderness or adnexal masses. Finally examination of the anus should include note of perianal skin tags or fissures that may be associated with inflammatory bowel disease or trauma.

Diagnostic Evaluation

Pelvic imaging is useful to evaluate for congenital causes of pain as well as the presence of ovarian masses. In most young adolescents and postpubertal females, transabdominal ultrasound is adequate to assess the appendix, uterus, and ovaries for evidence of a cyst, tumor, or obstruction. Transvaginal ultrasound is more sensitive for a patient who is pregnant to determine the location of the pregnancy, if there is a concern for ectopic pregnancy or spontaneous abortion. Doppler assessment may provide information about the vascular flow to the adnexa, but the presence of flow does not exclude ovarian torsion as the etiology for pain [4]. Three-dimensional ultrasound is also an effective imaging modality for Mullerian anomalies [5,6].

Magnetic resonance imaging (MRI) is the modality of choice for Mullerian anomalies and can also evaluate renal and spinal anomalies. Of note, a detailed protocol to assess the cervix and upper vagina can increase the sensitivity of evaluation of obstructive anomalies [7]. If there is a known congenital anomaly, such as unilateral renal agenesis or cloacal anomaly, MRI evaluation can determine the presence of a uterovaginal anomaly, including a transverse septum or a noncommunicating functioning uterine horn. If the imaging is normal, then the most likely etiology for secondary dysmenorrhea in adolescents is endometriosis. Due to expense, MRI should not be considered a first-line radiologic examination.

Computerized tomography (CT) may be ordered for patients presenting with acute pain to assess for appendicitis or nephrolithiasis. The scan may then demonstrate findings of an ovarian cyst, tumor, or tubo-ovarian abscess. Although there are findings on CT that may be associated with adnexal torsion including Fallopian tube thickening and uterine deviation to the affected side, it is not the preferred imaging technique for evaluation of adnexal torsion [8]. Due to the radiation exposure, it should not be considered a first-line radiologic examination for patients with concern for ovarian cysts, torsion, or uterine anomaly.

Laboratory evaluation for pelvic pain may include urine pregnancy test and urinalysis to evaluate for hematuria and urinary tract infection. A complete blood count will assess the white blood cell count and hematocrit for infection or anemia; the erythrocyte sedimentation rate may be useful as a marker of inflammation. For any patient with a positive urine pregnancy test, a blood type to assess for Rh status and quantitative human chorionic gonadotropin (hCG) should be performed. Serum tumor markers may be helpful to assess the likelihood of an ovarian malignancy, if imaging reveals an ovarian mass with solid elements or if the tumor is large. Epithelial malignancies in adolescence are rare and therefore tumor markers associated with non-epithelial ovarian cancer, such as serum hCG, inhibin, alpha fetoprotein (AFP), testosterone, and estradiol may be collected [9]. If there is concern for an obstruction with a known renal anomaly, a creatinine can assess for renal insufficiency. Finally, gonorrhea and chlamydia testing should be performed in any patient with a history of sexual activity by vaginal swab or urine testing.

Condition-specific Management Strategies

Primary Dysmenorrhea

Relief of primary dysmenorrhea is usually accomplished with the use of a nonsteroidal anti-inflammatory drug (NSAID) initiated at the onset and, ideally, 24 hours prior to the onset of menstruation if predictable, and continued for the first 2–3 days of the period. Prostaglandin inhibitors have been shown not only to decrease pain but also to decrease the amount of menstrual bleeding. Methods include naproxen, mefenamic acid, ibuprofen, or alternately celecoxib.

Primary dysmenorrhea may also be alleviated with combined oral, transvaginal, or transdermal contraceptives [10]. Combined contraceptive methods can be prescribed in a continuous versus cyclic manner to suppress pain and bleeding. Patients should be assessed for relative and absolute contraindications to treatment prior to initiation, including history of thrombosis, thrombophilia, hypertension, or migraines.

If estrogen is contraindicated, progesterone only methods are also effective, including depot medroxyprogesterone acetate (150 mg every 3 months), oral norethindrone or desogestrel, or the levonorgestrel intrauterine system. The etonogestrel implant may decrease pain but is less likely to achieve oligo or amenorrhea and has not been studied for its benefits in the management of dysmenorrhea.

A secondary cause of dysmenorrhea in adolescents should be suspected when the patient reports onset of symptoms at menarche or soon thereafter with worsening, debilitating pain, refractory to NSAIDs. When dysmenorrhea worsens and is not responding to a trial of a menstrual suppressive method, then an acquired cause of dysmenorrhea, including endometriosis, should be ruled out.

Endometriosis

Endometriosis, was long thought to be a condition primarily diagnosed during the third or fourth decade of life but has now been increasingly identified as a cause of dysmenorrhea in adolescents. Nevertheless, it remains an under-recognized entity in this age group, with the majority of adolescents having a - several year delay in diagnosis, often after seeing multiple specialists [11]. More than half of adolescents with pelvic pain not responding to menstrual suppression or NSAIDs and approximately half of those complaining of gastrointestinal and urinary symptoms are found to have endometriosis at laparoscopy [11,12]. Risk factors for the development of endometriosis include a family history of the disease, the presence of a congenital uterine anomaly, and early menarche [13,14].

Although ultrasonography and MRI have been used to identify endometriosis in older women, the gold standard for the diagnosis remains laparoscopy. Endometriomas are rare, and other ultrasound findings characteristic of severe endometriosis, including diminished ovarian or uterine mobility and tenderness, when exerting pressure on the adnexa or pouch of Douglas are not useful with transabdominal ultrasound. Chronic pain without improvement with a trial of menstrual suppression and NSAIDs in the absence of any other etiology is an indication for laparoscopic evaluation for endometriosis [11].

Operative Management

More than two-thirds of adolescents will be diagnosed with stage I endometriosis, although more severe disease has been reported [11,15]. The macroscopic appearance of endometriosis in adolescents differs from that found in adults, with white, clear, or red lesions; peritoneal defects; or scars being characteristic features (Figure 7B.1). Rarely, advanced blue or blackish lesions are identified [16,17]. To better

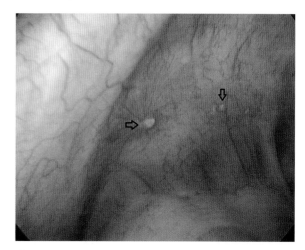

Figure 7B.1 Clear vesicular endometriosis lesions identified in the cul de sac during laparoscopy

visualize clear peritoneal lesions, the laparoscopic camera can be submerged in pooled irrigation fluid [17]. Ectopic endometriosis has been reported in previous abdominal scar sites, the lung, and the appendix. Approximately 30 percent of the time, the appendix can have early lesion involvement and be a continued source of pain for some females; therefore, diagnostic laparoscopy should include visualization of the appendix [17,18].

If a lesion is identified, it should be biopsied. Small lesions and adhesions can be ablated with cautery and CO_2 laser [17,18]. Peritoneal stripping to completely remove all endometriosis is controversial, especially in adolescents, and may not result in long-term symptomatic relief. When no lesions are visible, it is recommended to consider taking a random biopsy within the cul-de-sac, as this is a common location for early endometriosis lesions to be found.

Postoperative Management

Without ongoing medical treatment, endometriosis remains a chronic disease, likely to deteriorate in the future, with detrimental effects on fertility [16]. Therefore, surgery should be followed by long-term menstrual suppression to minimize disease progression. Although highly effective at suppression of endometriosis pain, the depo medroxyprogesterone acetate (DMPA) and gonadotropin-releasing hormone analogues (GnRH agonists) may impair bone mineralization, due to the complete follicular suppression and hypoestrogenism that they induce and are thus not a preferred long-term option in adolescents [20]. GnRH agonists should ideally be used with add-back therapy if treatment is prolonged beyond 6 months [16]. Danazol, a 17-alpha ethinyl-testosterone derivative, results in amenorrhea and is considered highly effective in the management of endometriosis, but it is also less favored among adolescents, due to unpleasant androgenic side effects, such as deepening of the voice and hirsutism. The levonorgestrel intrauterine device is now recommended by most scientific societies as a first-line long-acting contraceptive method in adolescence [21,22]. Evidence exists regarding its efficacy in the treatment of dysmenorrhea and endometriosis in adulthood and emerging data are suggesting that these management principles can be extrapolated to adolescents [23,24]. Another alternative may be a combined estrogen-progestin method, such as the combined oral contraceptive pill, which can be used continuously.

Endometriosis is associated with decreased physical and mental well-being. Close collaboration with psychologists, pain specialists, and social workers may be a valuable strategy to improve quality of life in young women with endometriosis [25]. With early identification and aggressive medical treatment, the progression of endometriosis can be minimized. For patients who are desiring pregnancy, early referral to a reproductive endocrinologist is appropriate if conception is delayed.

Congenital Anomalies

Incidence

The incidence of congenital anomalies of the reproductive tract ranges from 3.2 percent in asymptomatic fertile women undergoing tubal ligation to a high of 67 percent of patients with cloacal anomalies [26,27]. The absolute incidence of uterine and vaginal anomalies in adolescents with pelvic pain has not been established. The most common congenital anomalies identified include imperforate hymen, septate hymen, distal vaginal atresia, transverse vaginal septum, and obstructed uterine horn.

Operative Management

Imperforate Hymen

Imperforate hymen is most often a diagnosis that will be made at the time of puberty, when there is

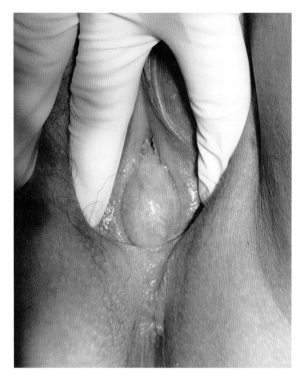

Figure 7B.2 The bulging imperforate hymen has a blue tinge

bulge of the hymen with proximal hematocolpos (Figure 7B.2). If mucocolpos is identified in infancy, surgical intervention is indicated if the mass effect causes urinary tract obstruction. It is recommended to remove as much hymenal tissue as is possible to prevent restenosis. Due to the risk of ascending infection with inadequate drainage, simple incision and drainage is not advised. For patients with hematocolpos, the hymenal tissue can be removed in a cruciate fashion or circumferentially to allow adequate vaginal width for tampon use, speculum examination, or coitus. If the hymenal tissue is very thin, the hymen may be resected with the cautery alone, followed by use of topical estrogen cream to aid wound healing. Otherwise, absorbable sutures are placed to approximate the mucosal edges to achieve hemostasis [28].

Transverse Vaginal Septum

Transverse septa are typically addressed surgically postpuberty when vaginal estrogenization improves healing. Using traction sutures on the distal vagina, a spinal needle may be advanced through the septum into the proximal vagina until hematocolpos contents are identified. Once the space is confirmed,

77

a transverse incision can then be made to enter the obstructed proximal vagina. All septal edges should be resected with care to avoid the bladder and rectum and the proximal vaginal mucosa should be anastomosed to the distal vaginal mucosa with interrupted absorbable sutures. In cases of a thick transverse septum (longer than 1 cm), it may be necessary to perform a Z plasty technique to prevent vaginal stenosis [29].

If a microperforation is present, there may not be a bulging effect and preoperative assessment of the septal depth may be limited. Vaginoscopy may be performed in these cases to identify the microperforation (Figure 7B.3). With the Seldinger technique, the surgeon may place a catheter balloon through the microperforation into the proximal vagina and then place gentle traction. If pyocolpos or ascending infection is present, broad spectrum antibiotics should be prescribed. If the septum is thick or very proximal, a combined abdominal perineal approach is advisable, so as to identify the level of obstruction proximally and guide the surgical approach from the perineum to allow resection of the septum at the appropriate level, thus avoiding injury to adjacent structures [30]. Postoperatively, a vaginal stent may minimize stenosis [28]. Adolescents post-resection of a high vaginal septum will need to start vaginal dilation within a few days postoperatively. The process of dilation should be guided by a physician, nurse, or physical therapist with expertise. Psychological support should be provided for both the patient and her family [30].

Obstructed Hemivagina

OHVIRA (obstructed hemivagina ipsilateral renal agenesis) is a variation of the transverse septum Due to uterine didelphys, typically only one hemivagina will be patent and one will be obstructed. When the obstructed hemivagina is distended, traction sutures may be placed and the location of the obstructed proximal vagina identified with the spinal needle technique. Care should be taken to remove all edges of the septum. When the septum is thick, it may be necessary to place a stent to minimize postoperative stenosis. Similar to the transverse septum, vaginoscopy can help to better visualize if a microperforation is present. Interrupted absorbable sutures should be used to approximate the vaginal mucosa of the proximal and distal vaginal tissues after the septum has been optimally excised.

Distal Vaginal Atresia

Distal vaginal atresia will typically present at puberty. There may be a bulge visualized at the perineum, but there is no evidence of the bluish tinge seen with an imperforate hymen (Figure 7B.4). A rectal exam to palpate the hematocolpos may determine the distance from the proximal vagina to the perineum. When the distance of the proximal vagina is less than 3 cm from the perineum, a simple pull through vaginoplasty should be performed. One can confirm the location of the

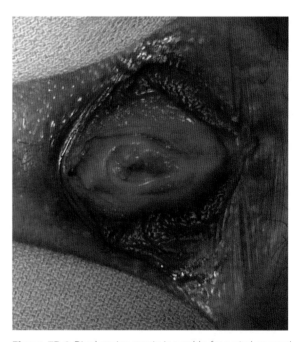

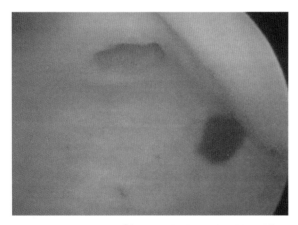

Figure 7B.3 Inspection of the vaginal wall reveals old blood from the obstructed hemivagina draining into the patent vagina in a patient with OHVIRA.

Figure 7B.4 Distal vagina atresia is notable for typical mucosal color at the introitus.

hematocolpos by using the spinal needle technique with serial traction sutures placed on the proximal vagina to facilitate mobilization. An incision may be extended transversely and septal tissues should be resected. After adequate mobilization, the upper vaginal mucosal edges are sewn to the introitus with interrupted absorbable suture. When the distance is farther than 3 cm, one may consider an interposition graft or recommend menstrual suppression until the patient is ready to dilate. She may be able to dilate the distal vaginal dimple preoperatively to decrease the septal thickness. With high distal atresia, placement of a postoperative vaginal stent and postoperative dilation are important to minimize stenosis [28].

Obstructed Uterine Horns

Patients with Mayer-Rokitansky-Kuster-Hauser (MRKH) or with a unicornuate uterus are at high risk for remnant uterine horns, which may contain functional endometrial cavities. These remnants may be excised laparoscopically with cautery or a vessel-sealing device. The remnants may be found from the midline to the lateral pelvic sidewalls. Uterine and renal anomalies are commonly associated; therefore, utmost care should be taken to avoid injuring aberrant urologic structures [28,31].

Cervical Atresia

One of the most challenging diagnoses is cervicovaginal agenesis. Menstrual suppression to alleviate pain can allow time for adequate preoperative patient counseling and operative planning. Definitive management includes removal of the remnant uterus, potentially laparoscopically. One may consider use of ureteral stents prior to starting the dissection to minimize the risk of ureteral injury.

Several reports describe attempts to anastomose the vagina directly to the uterus. Uterovaginal anastomosis involves resecting the obliterated cervix followed by anastomosis of the uterine isthmus to the upper vagina. There have been a few published cases of pregnancy after this procedure [32]. Due to the inability to recreate the muscular and immune properties innate to the cervix that typically protect the reproductive structures from ascending infections, there have also been cases of sepsis and death. The first few weeks and months are critical for stenosis. Although a second attempt for cervical recanalization can be performed following uterovaginal anastomosis, cases of relapses will most likely require a hysterectomy. Due to the high risk of complications, uterovaginal anastomoses is a controversial procedure [28].

Fertility

In the case of obstructive reproductive tract anomalies, the risk of endometriosis is significantly higher; therefore, the patient should be counseled that menstrual suppression may not only treat ongoing pelvic pain but also improve fertility outcomes [28,33].

Young girls with a unicornuate or didelphys uterus can be reassured that the live birthrate is at least 60 percent. There is a higher risk of cervical incompetence, second trimester miscarriage, preterm labor, abnormal placentation, and intrauterine growth restriction [34]. It is therefore advisable that women with a congenital uterine anomaly are carefully followed during their pregnancy with serial cervical measurements and growth scans by an experienced obstetrician.

Adnexal Cysts

Adnexal cysts are common and typically found with normal ovarian physiologic processes. If a cyst is identified by ultrasound; is small, simple, or hemorrhagic; and the patient does not have an acute abdomen, supportive management with pain medication is typically sufficient. Follow-up imaging will usually show resolution of the physiologic cyst [35]. Indications for surgical intervention include severe pain concerning for torsion or active intraperitoneal hemorrhage, imaging findings concerning for neoplasia (solid portions larger than 2 cm, multiple septae, size larger than 8 cm), or persistence with follow-up imaging [9].

Management

The goals of surgical intervention include alleviation of pain, removal of neoplastic tissue, and optimization of future fertility. Ovarian cysts in children and adolescents can be managed in a minimally invasive fashion with laparoscopy, with few exceptions. These exceptions include multiple prior abdominal surgeries or medical conditions that prevent them from tolerating a procedure laparoscopically [36,37]. Persistent and large symptomatic ovarian cysts should be removed laparoscopically if there are no concerning features for malignancy and tumor markers are negative [9,37]. Although ultrasound may confirm the presence of a cyst, it may not be possible to determine the cyst origin until intraoperative visualization. Whether the cyst originates from the ovary or the Fallopian tube, a simple cystectomy is typically sufficient. Cystectomy and ovarian preservation are recommended for benign neoplasia, including teratomas, serous cystadenomas, and mucinous cystadenomas. If there is high suspicion for a malignancy due to large solid components, ascites, or elevated tumor markers, then unilateral salpingooophorectomy is recommended with surgical staging [9,36,37]. In pediatric and adolescent patients with germ cell malignancies, the Children's Oncology Group staging also includes pelvic cytology from pelvic washings or ascites, peritoneal cavity inspection for and biopsy of peritoneal implants, palpation of pelvic lymph nodes with sampling of enlarged nodes, omental inspection and biopsy if lesions are identified, and inspection of the contralateral ovary [9,38]. If an epithelial malignancy is identified, then International Federation of Gynecology and Obstetrics (FIGO) staging is recommended [39].

Physiologic Cysts

For cysts that are found incidentally during another procedure, the surgeon may confirm that it is merely a functional follicle and when small, no intervention is necessary. Other functional cysts, such as hemorrhagic cysts, may be symptomatic, as is the case for an actively bleeding or expanding hemorrhagic ovarian cyst. In this situation, removal of the cyst wall and cauterizing the ovarian tissue bed is typically necessary to halt ongoing bleeding [37].

Adnexal Torsion

In cases of adnexal torsion, it is important to detorse the adnexa, ovary, and/or Fallopian tube. Even if the adnexal structures appear blue or black and there is concern for diminished viability, every attempt should be made to salvage these structures. Despite the necrotic appearance, detorsion may allow the ovary to regain function [40,41]. Adnexal structures may be detorsed and then observed for return of color [36,43]. In a recent study, children and adolescents with ovarian torsion underwent surgical detorsion and ovarian preservation, irrespective of intraoperative appearance. Subsequent ultrasounds demonstrated that 96.6 percent of ovaries recovered function [42].

When a cyst is present in the setting of torsion, if the cyst can be dissected easily, it should be removed to minimize risk of retorsion. In cases of a large adnexal cyst, it may be necessary to perform a cystectomy to achieve complete detorsion.

Oophoropexy

Whether or not to perform oophoropexy is controversial. Experienced surgeons may choose to perform an oophoropexy if the uteroovarian ligament is abnormally elongated. When one finds no evidence of an ovarian cyst, but torsion has resulted in significant edematous changes of the ovary and tube, this bulky adnexa may need to be pexed temporarily to allow swelling to resolve and minimize the risk of retorsion [44,45]. Bivalving to improve blood flow and to debulk the ovary may decrease the risk of retorsion [46]. In the situation of recurrent torsion or a solitary remaining ovary, oophoropexy with a permanent suture may minimize the risk of another torsion.

Postoperative Management

Depending on the underlying cyst pathology, the risk of recurrence may vary [9]. After detorsion, a follow-up ultrasound in 6 weeks to 3 months to assess recovery is reasonable. Hormonal suppression of ovulation may be warranted [37,42,44,45]. A follow-up ultrasound in 1 year is typically adequate to assess for recurrence for benign ovarian tumors [9].

Conclusion

A wide variety of pathology may lead to pelvic pain in adolescence. Most girls will experience some degree of discomfort during menstruation, which will be relieved with simple analgesics. When the pain is severe or refractory to usual treatment, a secondary cause for dysmenorrhea, such as endometriosis should be sought. Congenital Mullerian anomalies causing obstruction will typically present around the time of menarche, either with severe dysmenorrhea or cyclical pelvic pain. Surgical management goals include restoring the passage of menstruation, while optimizing future fertility. Functional ovarian cysts are common, mostly due to the higher incidence of anovulatory cycles in the first years after menarche. Cautious observation is usually advisable, but surgical intervention may be required in case of acute hemorrhage, torsion, or persistence. Prevention of cyst recurrences and progression of endometriosis is usually achieved through menstrual suppression.

References

1. Suvitie PA, Hallamaa MK, Matomaki JM et al. Prevalence of pain symptoms suggestive of endometriosis among Finnish adolescent girls (teen maps study). *J Pediatr Adolesc Gynecol* 2016; **29**: 97–103.

2. Zannoni L, Giorgi M, Spagnolo E et al. Dysmenorrhea, absenteeism from school and symptoms suspicious for endometriosis in adolescents. *J Pediatr Adolesc Gynecol* 2014; **27**: 258–65.

3. Iacovides S, Avidon I, Baker F. What we know about primary dysmenorrhea today: a critical review. *Hum Rep Update* 2015; **21**: 762–78.

4. Naiditch J, Barsness K. The positive and negative predictive value of transabdominal color Doppler ultrasound for diagnosing ovarian torsion in pediatric patients. *J Pediatr Surg* 2013; **48**: 1283–87.

5. Deutch T, Abuhamad A. The role of 3-dimensional ultrasonography and magnetic resonance imaging in the diagnosis of mullerian duct anomalies: a review of the literature. *J Ultrasound Med* 2008; **27**: 413–23.

6. Caliskan E, Ozkan S, Cakiroglu Y et al. Diagnostic accuracy of real-time 3D sonography in the diagnosis of congenital mullerian anomalies in high-risk patients with respect to the phase of the menstrual cycle. *J Clin Ultrasound* 2010; **38**: 123–27.

7. Saleem S. MR imaging diagnosis of uterovaginal anomalies: current state of the art. *Radiographics* 2003; **23**: e13.

8. Lee J, Park S, Shin S. Value of intra-adnexal and extra-adnexal computed tomographic imaging features diagnosing torsion of adnexal tumor. *J Comput Assist Tomogr* 2009; **33**: 872–76.

9. Amies Oelschlager A, Gow K, Morse C et al. Management of large ovarian neoplasms in pediatric and adolescent females. *J Pediatr Adolesc Gynecol* 2016; **29**: 88–94.

10. Davies A, Westhoff C, O'Connell K et al. Oral contraceptives for dysmenorrhea in adolescent girls: a randomized trial. *Obstet Gynecol* 2005; **106**: 97–104.

11. Dun E, Kho K, Morozov V et al. Endometriosis in adolescents. *J Soc Laparoendoscopic Surg* 2015; **19**: 1–8.

12. Greene R, Stratton P, Cleary S et al. Diagnostic experience among 1334 women reporting surgically diagnosed endometriosis. *Fertil Steril* 2009; **91**: 32–39.

13. Dalsgaard T, Hjordt Hansen MV, Hartwell D et al. Reproductive prognosis in daughters of women with and without endometriosis. *Hum Repr* 2013; **28**: 2284–88.

14. Nnoaham K, Webster P, Kumbang J et al. Is early age at menarche a risk factor for endometriosis? A systematic review and meta-analysis of case-control studies. *Fertil Steril* 2012; **98**: 702–12.

15. Reese KA, Reddy S, Rock JA. Endometriosis in an adolescent population: the Emory experience. *J Pediatr Adolesc Gynecol* 1996; **9**: 125.

16. American College of Obstetricians and Gynecologists. ACOG Committee opinion Number 310. Endometriosis in adolescents. *Obstet Gynecol* 2005; **105**: 921–27.

17. Laufer M, Sanfilippo J, Rose G. Adolescent endometriosis: diagnosis and treatment approaches. *J Pediatr Adolesc Gynecol* 2003; **16**: S3–11.

18. Doyle J, Missmer S, Laufer M. The effect of combined surgical-medical intervention on the progression of endometriosis in an adolescent and young adult population. *J Pediatr Adolesc Gynecol* 2009; **22**: 257–63.

19. Brosens I, Gordts S, Benagiano G. Endometriosis in adolescents is a hidden, progressive and severe disease that deserves attention, not just compassion. *Hum Reprod* 2013; **28**: 2026–31.

20. Lara-Torre E, Edwards C, Pearlman S et al. Bone mineral density in adolescent females using depot medroxyprogesterone acetate. *J Pediatr Adolesc Gynecol* 2004; **17**: 17–21.

21. American College of Obstetricians and Gynecologists Committee on Adolescent Health Care Long-acting Reversible Contraception Working Group. ACOG Committee opinion Number 539. Adolescents and long-acting reversible contraception: implants and intrauterine devices. *Obstet Gynecol* 2012; **120**: 983–88.

22. Ott M, Sucato G and Committee on Adolescence. American Academy of Pediatrics. Technical report: contraception for adolescents. *Pediatrics* 2014; **134**: e1257–81.

23. Abou-Setta A, Houston B, Al-Inany H et al. Levonorgestrel-releasing intrauterine device (LNG-IUD) for symptomatic endometriosis following surgery. *Cochrane Database Syst Rev* 2013; Jan 31.

24. Yoost J, LaJoie A, Hertweck P et al. Use of the LNG IUS in adolescents with endometriosis. *J Pediatr Adolesc Gynecol* 2013; **26**: 120–24.

25. De Graaff A, D'Hooghe T, Dunselman G et al. The significant effect of endometriosis on physical, mental and social wellbeing: results from an international cross-sectional survey. *Hum Reprod* 2013; **28**: 2677–85.

26. Simon C, Martinez I, Pardo F et al. Mullerian defects in women with normal reproductive outcome. *Fertil Steril* 1991; **56**: 1192–93.

27. Breech L. Gynecologic concerns in patients with cloacal anomaly. *Semin Pediatr Surg* 2016; **25**: 90–95.

28. Dietrich J, Miller D, Quint E. Obstructive reproductive tract anomalies. *J Pediatr Adolesc Gynecol* 2014; **27**: 396–402.

29. Wierrani F, Boner K, Spangler B et al. "Z"-plasty of the transverse vaginal septum using Garcia's procedure and the Grunberger modification. *Fertil Steril* 2003; **79**: 608–12.

30. Williams C, Nakhal R, Hall-Craggs M et al. Transverse vaginal septae: management and long-term outcomes. *Brit J Obstet Gynecol* 2014; **121**: 1653–58.

31. Will M, Marsh C, Smorgick N et al. pearls: laparoscopic removal of uterine remnants with Mayer-Rokitansky-Kuster-Hauser syndrome. *J Pediatr Adolesc Gynecol* 2013; **26**: 224–27.

32. Deffarges J, Haddad B, Musset R et al. Utero-vaginal anastomosis in women with uterine cervix atresia: long-term follow-up and reproductive performance. A study of 18 cases. *Hum Reprod* 2001; **16**: 1722–25.

33. Silveira S, Laufer M. Persistence of endometriosis after correction of an obstructed reproductive tract anomaly. *J Pediatr Adolesc Gynecol* 2013; **26**: e93–94.

34. Grimbizis G, Camus M, Tarlatzis B et al. linical implications of uterine malformations and hysteroscopic treatment results. *Hum Reprod Update* 2001; **7**: 161–74.

35. Strickland J. Ovarian cysts in neonates, children and adolescents. *Curr Opin Obstet Gynecol* 2002; **14**: 459–65.

36. Rieger M, Santos X, Sangi-Haghpeykar H et al. Laparoscopic outcomes for pelvic pathology in children and adolescent among patients presenting to the pediatric and adolescent gynecology service. *J Pediatr Adolesc Gynecol* 2015; **28**: 157–62.

37. Kirkham Y, Kives S. Ovarian cysts in adolescents: medical and surgical management. *Adolesc Med State Art Rev* 2012; **23**: 178–91.

38. Billmire D, Vinocur F, Rescorla B et al. Outcome and staging evaluation in malignant germ cell tumors of the ovary in children and adolescents: An intergroup study. *J Pediatr Surg* 2004; **39**: 424–29.

39. Pecorelli S, Benedet J, Creasman W et al. FIGO staging of gynecologic cancer. 1994–1997 FIGO Committee on Gynecologic Oncology. International Federation of Gynecology and Obstetrics. *Int J Gynaecol Obstet* 1999; **65**: 243–49.

40. Eckler K, Laufer M, Perlman S. Conservative management of bilateral asynchronous adnexal torsion with necrosis in a prepubertal girl. *J Pediatr Surg* 2000; **35**: 1248–51.

41. Galinier P, Carfagna I, Delsol M et al. Ovarian torsion. Management and ovarian prognosis: a report of 45 cases. *J Pediatr Surg* 2009; **44**: 1759–65.

42. Santos X, Cass D, Dietrich J. Outcome following detorsion of torsed adnexa in children. *J Pediatr Adolesc Gynecol* 2015; **28**: 136–38.

43. Karayalcin R, Ozcan S, Ozyer S et al. Conservative laparoscopic management of adnexal torsion. *J Turk Ger Gynecol Assoc* 2011; **12**: 4–8.

44. Ashwal E, Hiersch L, Krissi H et al. Characteristics and management of ovarian torsion in premenarchal compared with postmenarchal patients. *Obstet Gynecol* 2015; **126**: 514–20.

45. Rossi B, Ference E, Zurakowski D et al. The clinical presentation and surgical management of adnexal torsion in the pediatric and adolescent population. *J Pediatr Adolesc Gynecol* 2012; **25**: 109–13.

46. Styer A, Laufer M. Ovarian bivalving after detorsion. *Fertil Steril* 2002; **77**: 1053–55.

Primary Amenorrhea in Pediatric and Adolescent Gynecology Practice
Clinical Evaluation

Naomi S. Crouch and Lisa Allen

Presentation and Definition

Ninety-eight percent of young women reach menarche by age 15, indicating that while amenorrhea is reasonably rare, it remains a common reason for referral to a pediatric and adolescent gynecologist. In the pubertal time line, menarche is usually achieved within 3 years of the onset of thelarche. While the age of onset of thelarche has declined, the age of menarche has remained relatively stable. In a menstrual cycle, gonadotropin releasing hormone (GnRH) is released from the hypothalamus to the anterior pituitary, which in turn releases follicle stimulating hormone (FSH) and luteinizing hormone (LH). These act on the ovary, which responds by allowing maturation of ova, and the subsequent menstrual cycle. The achievement of menses in puberty, therefore, requires a functioning hypothalamic-pituitary-ovarian axis, the presence of a uterus as well as an intact and non-obstructed outflow tract.

Two-thirds of women will have a sexual maturity rating of IV according to Tanner stages, for both breast and pubic hair at the time of menarche (see Table 8A.1). While traditionally the definition of primary amenorrhea was the absence of menses by age 16, recognition of the usual pubertal milestones has resulted in revised recommendations. Evaluation for primary amenorrhea should therefore be initiated for the following criteria [1]:

1. No menses by age of 15 regardless of the presence of normal growth and development of secondary sexual characteristics
2. No menses within 3 years of thelarche
3. No menses by age 14 in the absence of growth spurt or development of secondary sexual characteristics
4. No menses by age 14 with signs of hirsutism or a history or examination of excessive exercise or eating disorder

Table 8A.1 Sexual Maturity Ratings for Girls

Stage	Breast	Pubic Hair
1	Elevation of papilla only	No pubic hair
2	Elevation of the breast and papilla, areolar diameter enlarges (breast bud)	Sparse, downy hair, straight or only slightly curly primarily along labia
3	Further enlargement of breast and areola, no separation of contours	Darker, coarser, curly hair with more spread
4	Secondary mound consisting of the projection of the areola and papilla above level of breast	Adult hair type spreads over the mon pubis but not the inner surface of thighs
5	Mature breast with recession of areola to general contour of the breast	Adult-type hair in quality and quantity, spreads to inner surface of thighs

5. No menses at any age with symptoms suggestive of an outflow tract obstruction, such as cyclic abdominal pain or an abdominal mass

The approach to evaluation of an individual with primary amenorrhea is to first determine which broad category is the likely etiology for the amenorrhea, then to determine the specific diagnosis. Hypergonadotropic hypogonadism is the most common category at 48.5 percent, followed by Mullerian agenesis 16.2 percent, gonadotropin deficiency 8.3 percent, and constitutional delay 6 percent [2].

The common causes of primary amenorrhea are listed in Table 8A.2.

History

As with any reproductive health care visit, the history from the adolescent should be structured with

Table 8A.2 Causes of Primary Amenorrhea

Category	Diagnosis
Increased serum gonadotropins (hypergonadotropic hypogonadism)	• Premature Ovarian Insufficiency • XX or XY gonadal dysgenesis • Turner Syndrome • Irradiation/cytotoxic therapy • Autoimmune/infectious/galactosemia/Fragile X
Normal or low serum gonadotropins (hypogonadotropic hypogonadism or eugonadotropic hypogonadism)	• Constitutional Delay • Hypopituitarism • Panhypopituitarism • Isolated gonadotropin deficiency • Isolated GH deficiency • Kallman syndrome (with anosmia) • Hypothalamic dysfunction • Chronic illness (obstructive sleep apnea, HIV, IBD, celiac disease, CF, renal disease, Fe deposition with transfusion dependent hemoglobinopathies) • Eating disorders/excess exercise/stress • CNS tumors/lesions/malformations • Hypothyroidism • Hyperprolactinemia, i.e., adenoma, medication • Syndromes with Hypo-hypo Prader-Willi, Lawrence-Moon syndrome, Bardet Bield
Other conditions	• Anatomic Abnormalities (Mullerian agenesis, cervical agenesis, transverse septum, imperforate hymen) • Androgen insensitivity syndrome • Noonan's

sensitivity and reassurance of confidentiality. A full pubertal time line should be established, determining the ages of growth spurt, thelarche, and adrenarche if these have occurred.

It is important to inquire about sexual activity, consensual or nonconsensual, and use of contraception as pregnancy must be within the differential diagnosis of amenorrhea at any age, even if the presentation is of primary amenorrhea. A sexual history should always be enquired about in the absence of a parent or caregiver.

The adolescent should be questioned regarding associated symptoms: cyclic abdominal pain, weight loss, disordered eating, excess exercise, symptoms of hypothyroidism, galactorrhea, headaches, anosmia, hirsutism, or virilization. An interview instrument

such as the HEADSS (Home, Education/Employment, Activities, Drugs, Sexuality, Suicide/Depression) assessment [3] is recommended during any encounter with an adolescent. Completion of such screening may reveal sources of stress that the adolescent is experiencing. A thorough medical and surgical history should be included.

In constitutional delay of puberty, there is generally a family history of at least one parent who experienced late onset of puberty.

Clinical Findings

A general assessment should form part of the physical examination, in particular documenting both height and weight, allowing calculation of the body mass index. Height should be plotted on a standardized growth curve. Sexual development can be ascertained by determining the sexual maturing ratings (SMR) of both breast and pubic hair (see Table 8A.1). Short stature and absence of secondary sexual characteristics suggest either hypogonadotropic or hypergonadotropic hypogonadism as an etiology of delayed puberty. A discrepancy in SMR of breast and pubic hair should lead to the suspicion of a chromosomal anomaly, for example, with Turner's syndrome adrenarche will occur without gonadarche, in cases of complete androgen insensitivity syndrome (CAIS), thelarche will occur without pubarche.

The patency of the outflow tract should be determined. An imperforate hymen is visible as a bluish, bulging membrane at the introitus most visible with Valsalva maneuver. Other obstructive anomalies may not be visible at the introitus such as in the presence of a vaginal septum. In long-standing cases of outflow tract obstruction, a palpable abdominal mass may be present due to the cryptomenorrhea. An abdominal mass could also represent an ovarian or adrenal tumor.

Specific features of the various differential diagnoses may be evident on examination. With Turner's syndrome, in addition to the short stature, other features include retrognathia, a high arched palate, a wide carrying angle, a low hairline, and low set ears with a webbed neck. Young women with polycystic ovarian syndrome may be overweight, have signs of clinical hyperandrogenism such as acne or hirsutism, and demonstrate acanthosis. Bradycardia, lanugo hair, low blood pressure, or signs of bulimia may be present with an eating disorder. The thyroid should be palpated for enlargement or nodules. Fundoscopy in the presence of a pituitary tumor might show bulging optic discs, and bilateral temporal hemianopia could be detected on visual field testing.

Initial Investigations

The information gathered from your physical examination and history will determine the most appropriate initial investigations. Any suspicion of pregnancy must be ruled out as a first step usually with a urine or serum BHCG.

Gonadotropin levels (FSH and LH) along with estradiol can be used to stratify into conditions of hypergonadotropic hypogonadism or those with a eugonadotropic/hypogonadotropic state. Of note in order to diagnose premature ovarian insufficiency (POI), two measurements of FSH > 25 IU/L more than 4 weeks apart are necessary [4]. If POI is confirmed, a karyotype, Fragile X premutation and adrenal and thyroid antibodies should be ordered to determine the cause.

Where clinical hyperandrogenism is evident, DHEAS, total and/or free testosterone should be assessed. Ovarian imaging can be deferred in adolescents for the diagnosis of polycystic ovarian syndrome (PCOS), although it may be indicated if there is concern of a virilizing ovarian tumor, as there is no compelling criteria for polycystic ovarian morphology in adolescents [5]. If serum DHEAS is elevated, a 17 hydroxy-progesterone acetate level will screen for late onset 21 hydroxylase deficiency.

Constitutional delay of puberty is differentiated from other etiologies of hypogonadotropic hypogonadism largely with time, as pubertal development will occur at ages 16–18. Basal LH and FSH levels as well as stimulated levels will overlap. Prolactin is usually included in early laboratory investigations. Suspicion of thyroid dysfunction should prompt inclusion of a thyroid stimulating hormone (TSH). An MRI of the pituitary is indicated with significantly elevated prolactin levels and/or in the presence of neurologic symptoms.

While an imperforate hymen can be diagnosed clinically, other outflow obstruction anomalies require imaging studies. The usual first-line imaging in adolescents with Mullerian anomalies is 2D ultrasound. Magnetic resonance imaging is confirmatory and considered the gold standard in this age group [6]. If a uterus is absent, a karyotype will be indicated to differentiate MRKH syndrome from CAIS, although clues to the latter include an absence of pubic and axillary hair.

Making the Diagnosis

Anatomical Causes

When all blood test results are normal, and secondary sexual characteristics are present, it is likely that there is an anatomical reason for the primary amenorrhea, as discussed earlier. Further imaging will allow detection of the anomaly, and as mentioned MRI is the gold standard [7]. It will give clear information regarding the presence of a uterus and endometrium, and the level of any obstruction. It will also give information on the number and location of the kidneys and ureters. With significant advances in MRI and with increased radiological expertise, there is no indication for a laparoscopy and hysteroscopy in making the diagnosis of a Mullerian anomaly.

Imperforate Hymen

An imperforate hymen is usually recognized as a blueish bulge seen on perineal inspection, with the obstructed menstrual flow visible behind the hymenal membrane. It is treated by a cruciate incision, which minimizes the chance of vaginal stenosis, and drainage of the accumulated blood. It is rarely associated with any other Mullerian or renal anomalies, and usually no further treatment is needed.

Transverse Septum

In contrast to an imperforate hymen, a transverse vaginal septum is rare, and the level of the blockage most commonly occurs from the middle third of the vagina upward toward the cervix. An MRI will give information regarding the level and thickness of the septum. Treatment is surgical excision of the septum and anastomosing the upper and lower parts of the vagina. This used to involve a combined abdomino-perineal approach, but now it can be performed with minimal-access surgery either vaginally or combined with laparoscopy [8]. This is complex surgery and should only be performed in a center of excellence by a team with both advanced laparoscopic and pediatric and adolescent gynecological skills.

Such surgery takes time to arrange, and the patient should be offered menstrual suppression from the time of diagnosis to prevent more menstrual obstruction. Suppression can be achieved with the use of continuous hormonal contraceptives, depo-medroxy-progesterone acetate, and rarely requires GnRH agonist. Endometriosis may have developed as a result of the obstruction, but this usually resolves once the obstruction is treated. Postoperatively, vaginal dilation should be performed to reduce the chance of stenosis to the newly connected vagina.

Cervical Agenesis

Cervical agenesis, the lack of development of the cervix, most often with the absence of the upper vagina, is an especially rare Mullerian anomaly occurring with an incidence of 1:80,000. This anomaly should be referred to centers of excellence for management. Menstrual suppression should be initiated as earlier discussed for transverse vaginal septums for symptom management.

Mayer-Rokitansky-Kuster-Hauser Syndrome

Approximately 1:5000 girls will have congenital absence of the upper vagina and uterus, also known as Mayer-Rokitansky-Kuster-Hauser (MRKH, or Rokitansky syndrome). The cause is unknown although both genetic factors and environmental factors have been postulated. The ovaries are present so other pubertal development proceeds normally. An ultrasound usually shows the lack of a uterus, which can be confirmed with MRI. There may be associated renal anomalies that can be detected by MRI. Occasionally this may present as part of a syndrome with Mullerian, renal, and cervical spine anomalies (MuRCS).

The mainstay of treatment is for development of a vagina sufficient for comfortable penetrative intercourse. Vaginal dilator therapy is effective for up to 85 percent of cases and carries minimal risks. This is the first-choice treatment [9]. For those for whom vaginal dilation is not effective, the laparoscopic Vecchietti procedure or Davydov procedure is indicated. Complex vaginoplasty surgery such as bowel or skin vaginoplasties carry significant morbidities and long-term risks and are not indicated for MRKH. They should not be offered until other options have been fully explored.

Until recently, the main options for fertility were for IVF using the individual's ova, via surrogacy, or for adoption. Surrogacy is legal in the UK but is not in all countries and can be a complex financial and emotional journey.

The development of uterine transplant surgery with successful pregnancies has given hope to many women with MRKH. However, this is still at a research stage

and the amount of extensive surgery for both donor and recipient should be fully appreciated.

While the treatment for developing a functional vagina is straightforward, the psychological impact of the diagnosis is immense and should not be underestimated. Many barriers may exist between the female achieving an increased vaginal length, and psychological support is essential. The implications for sexual function and for fertility and partnerships need to be explored. Dilation to the vagina should only begin when the patient is ready, which is rarely at the time of diagnosis.

Further details regarding MRKH may be found in Chapter 8C.

Endocrine Axis Causes

Hypogondadotrophic Hypogonadism

When FSH and LH levels are low, with no secondary sexual characteristics, there is a lack of GnRH being released from the hypothalamus. An ultrasound scan will show normal ovaries and uterus, but these will be of prepubertal dimensions. Some girls may present as a result of constitutional delay. There may be a family history of this. However, it should be considered a diagnosis of exclusion before reassuring the family.

There are many etiologies for hypogonadotrophic hypogonadism, such as chronic illness or eating disorders. It may also be part of rare syndromes such as Kallman syndrome, which includes anosmia or a genetic syndrome such as Prader-Willi syndrome. A comprehensive summary appears in Table 8A.2.

Puberty may be induced using gradually increasing amounts of estrogen patches and should be supervised by an endocrinology specialist or pediatric gynecologist experienced in pubertal induction [10]. Progestogen is added once menstruation starts, which is usually 2–3 years into the process.

Assisted conception is usually required, consisting of the ovaries being stimulated with pulses of FSH and LH. This care is offered within specialist fertility services and should be supervised to minimize the chance of multiple pregnancies.

PCOS

Polycystic ovary syndrome encompasses a wide range of presentations, but it is broadly considered to occur when two of the following are present: hyperandrogenism, infrequent menstrual bleeding and anovulation, or polycystic appearance to the ovaries. As the ovaries commonly display a multicystic pattern in adolescence, an ultrasound scan is not helpful in making the diagnosis at this age. With the ever-increasing accuracy of ultrasound, criteria for the current classification continue to be debated [11]. The majority of individuals will present with secondary amenorrhea, but occasionally primary amenorrhea is associated with the more marked variants of PCOS. Further details regarding PCOS appear in Chapter 8B. It is difficult to make the diagnosis of PCOS within 2 years of menarche, and many of the symptoms of PCOS are similar to normal symptoms of adolescence (irregular menses, acne).

Treatment would be as for adult women with PCOS to encourage weight loss as appropriate, and to ensure regular menstruation, usually with the oral contraceptive pill, patch, or ring. Evidence suggests that this approach leads to an improvement in quality of life for those with PCOS [12].

For those presenting with primary amenorrhea, the more severe congenital adrenal hyperplasia (CAH) needs to be excluded, by checking a 17 hydroxyprogesterone blood level. Such cases would be managed with an endocrinologist.

Primary Ovarian Insufficiency

Primary ovarian insufficiency (POI) is a rare condition in adolescents, although it occurs in approximately 1 percent of women under age 40. It may present with primary amenorrhea and varies as to whether the individual will have started puberty spontaneously, or with no signs of secondary sexual characteristics at all. FSH and LH levels will be persistently raised, with a corresponding low estrogen level. The uterus will have a prepubertal morphology. Up to 80 percent of girls will have no identifiable cause, but inborn errors of metabolism, autoimmune etiology, or Fragile X syndrome may be responsible for some cases, and a chromosome assessment should identify the latter. Management would be induction or continuation of puberty using estrogen, which should be guided by an experienced endocrinologist or pediatric gynecologist.

Disorders of Sex Development

Approximately 1:5000 girls are born with a disorder of sex development (DSD). Presentation may occur antenatally, when chromosomal analysis of the baby does not match the ultrasound appearance; at birth with atypical genitalia; or during childhood with an inguinal hernia in a girl, which proves to be the testes traveling toward the labioscrotal folds. In addition, adolescents may present with primary amenorrhea. Family details should be carefully noted, as it may become apparent that other younger siblings in the family also have a DSD. Once a diagnosis is suspected, care should be offered by an experienced multidisciplinary team with the core group consisting of a pediatric endocrinologist, gynecologist, psychologist, pediatric surgeon, or urologist [13]. Access to other team members such as a geneticist, radiologist, and biochemist should be available as needed.

Care should be taken regarding the use of terminology that patients and families find acceptable, and access to peer group support should be offered. Transition between pediatric to adult services may take several years but should be individualized to allow ongoing access to the lifelong care that those with DSDs require. Psychological support is an essential part of care for individuals with DSD diagnoses and should be organized for young women and families.

Androgen Insensitivity Syndrome

Complete androgen insensitivity syndrome (CAIS) has an incidence of approximately 1:40,000 births and arises as a result of a mutation on the androgen receptor (AR). The AR governs the virilization of the genitalia, and without activation, the baby will have normal external female appearance, despite a 46XY karyotype. As the gonads are functioning testes and produce Mullerian inhibiting substance (MIS), there are no internal Mullerian structures such as uterus or upper vagina, but the individual will have gone through spontaneous puberty from conversion of androgens to estrogen. Current management recommends gonadectomy to be performed once puberty is completed, around age 18 or 19 due to the small risk of gonadoblastoma development and lack of ability to monitor reliably [14]. This would then mean the patient should be taking hormone replacement therapy until age 50. Vaginal dilator therapy should be offered for the development of a vagina that allows comfortable penetrative intercourse, but the patient should choose the timing of this.

Gonadal Dysgenesis

In contrast to CAIS, those with 46XY gonadal dysgenesis will not have functioning gonads that allow a spontaneous puberty and may therefore present with no signs of secondary sexual characteristics. However, this also means that the gonads were not able to initiate the usual Wolfian Duct proliferation, and instead the internal structures will be a uterus and upper vagina, connecting to the normal lower vagina and female perineum.

The dysgenetic gonads carry a considerable (30 percent) risk of gonadoblastoma and therefore removal at the time of diagnosis is recommended. As for those with CAIS, hormone replacement therapy will be indicated until age 50 but would also need to be utilized to induce puberty. Again, this should be under the care of an experienced endocrinologist or pediatric gynecologist.

Further details regarding DSD are available in Chapter 8D.

Turner's Syndrome

Turner's syndrome (TS) occurs with an incidence of 1:2500 births. Fifty percent will have a complete absence of 1 X chromosome (45X0), while 35 percent to 45 percent will have mosaicism in their karyotype; the remaining will have a structurally abnormal X chromosome. The presence of a Y-containing fragment occurs in 5 percent. Similar to gonadal dysgenesis previously discussed, individuals with a Y-containing karyotype require gonadectomy for prevention of gonadoblastoma. Growth failure in girls with TS, due to the effect on the SHOX gene, usually starts early in life, by age 1.5; half of TS girls will have a height less than the 5th percentile. Growth hormone therapy is often considered to increase ultimate adult height under the direction of a pediatric endocrinologist. When diagnosed, investigations should occur for associated medical conditions most commonly renal (horseshoe kidney, malrotation) and cardiac (bicuspid aortic valve, coarctation of the aorta). If TS presents with the absence of pubertal development, pubertal induction should be instituted with the goals of the smooth acquisition of secondary sexual characteristics, optimizing psychosocial development, as well as developing and maintaining bone health. Unopposed estrogen is initiated first, at small doses and increased incrementally over several years. Progesterone is introduced when vaginal bleeding occurs or after 2 to 3 years of unopposed estrogen

therapy. Those with TS require lifelong care, with annual blood tests recommended to screen for other endocrine conditions, such as diabetes. Hypertension affects up to 50 percent of patients and needs to be treated aggressively to reduce cardiovascular risks such as aortic dissection. Additional tests such as cardiac MRI will help screen for aortic root dilation, and regular hearing tests to detect sensorineural deafness.

As with other DSDs, those with TS should be offered information regarding peer support groups and social media.

Conclusions

While primary amenorrhea remains rare, the causes are varied and a systematic approach will help elucidate any underlying condition. Girls and their families may present to any general gynecologist as well as those specialized in pediatric and adolescent care, and some understanding of potential diagnoses is essential. Stigma and shame have often surrounded some rarer conditions such as DSDs, and a sensitivity but honesty and openness regarding the diagnosis is needed. Psychological support is often under promoted by clinical services but remains a mandatory part of care for those with a DSD. Finally, peer support should be offered, with many excellent websites and social media groups now available to offer advice and guidance to those with more unusual conditions.

References

1. American College of Obstetricians and Gynecologists. ACOG Committee opinion Number 310. Menstruation in girls and adolescents: using the menstrual cycle as a vital sign. *Obstetrics and gynecology* 2015; **126**: e143–46.

2. Reindollar RH, Byrd JR, McDonough PG. Delayed sexual development: a study of 252 patients. *American Journal of Obstetrics and Gynecology* 1981; **140**: 371–80.

3. Cohen E, Mackenzie RG, Yates GL. HEADSS, a psychosocial risk assessment instrument: implications for designing effective intervention programs for runaway youth. *The Journal of Adolescent Health: Official Publication of the Society for Adolescent Medicine* 1991; **12**: 539–44.

4. European Society for Human Reproduction and Embryology Guideline Group on POI, Webber L, Davies M, Anderson RESHRE Guideline: management of women with premature ovarian insufficiency. *Human Reproduction* 2016; **31**: 926–37.

5. Witchel SF, Oberfield S, Rosenfield RL et al. The diagnosis of polycystic ovary syndrome during adolescence. *Hormone Research in Pediatrics* 2015; **83**: 376–89.

6. Grimbizis GF, Di Spiezio Sardo A, Saravelos SH et al. The Thessaloniki ESHRE/ESGE consensus on diagnosis of female genital anomalies. *Gynecological Surgery* 2016; **13**: 1–16.

7. Hall-Craggs MA, Kirkham A, Creighton SM. Renal and urological abnormalities occurring with Mullerian anomalies. *Journal of Pediatric Urology* 2013; **9**: 27–32.

8. Williams CE, Nakhal RS, Hall-Craggs MA et al. Transverse vaginal septae: management and long-term outcomes. *BJOG: An International Journal of Obstetrics and Gynecology* 2014; **121**: 1653–58.

9. Gargollo PC, Cannon GM Jr., Diamond DA et al. Should progressive perineal dilation be considered first line therapy for vaginal agenesis? *The Journal of Urology* 2009; **182**: 1882–89.

10. Royal College of Obstetricians and Gynecologists Scientific Impact Paper No. 40. Sex steroid treatment for pubertal induction and replacement in the adolescent girl. 2013. www.rcog.org.uk.

11. Dewailly D. Diagnostic criteria for PCOS: Is there a need for a rethink? *Best Practice & Research. Clinical Obstetrics & Gynecology* 2016 Nov; **37**: 5–11.

12. Dokras A, Sarwer DB, Allison KC et al. Weight loss and lowering androgens predict improvements in health-related quality of life in women with PCOS. *The Journal of Clinical Endocrinology and Metabolism* 2016; **101**: 2966–74.

13. Hughes IA, Houk C, Ahmed SF et al. Consensus statement on management of intersex disorders. *Archives of Disease in Childhood* 2006; **91**: 554–63.

14. Deans R, Creighton SM, Liao LM et al. Timing of gonadectomy in adult women with complete androgen insensitivity syndrome (CAIS): patient preferences and clinical evidence. *Clinical Endocrinology* 2012; **76**: 894–98.

Chapter 8B

Primary Amenorrhea in Pediatric and Adolescent Gynecology Practice
Endocrine Causes of Primary Amenorrhea

Adam Balen and Gerard S. Conway

Introduction

The endocrine causes of primary amenorrhea may result from abnormalities in the development of the ovaries, a disturbance of the normal endocrinological events of puberty or of the hypothalamic-pituitary-ovarian axis. Overall it is estimated that endocrine disorders account for approximately 25 percent of cases of primary amenorrhea [1,2].

The failure to menstruate by age 16 in the presence of normal secondary sexual development, or age 14 in the absence of secondary sexual characteristics warrants investigation. This distinction helps differentiate reproductive tract anomalies from gonadal quiescence and gonadal failure. Or in other words, to differentiate between estrogen replete and estrogen deficient states. A listing of the causes of primary amenorrhea is shown in Table 8B.1.

Secondary amenorrhea is the absence of menstruation of more than 6 months duration and may be temporary or permanent. Any cause of secondary amenorrhea may also cause primary amenorrhea. For example, weight loss, polycystic ovary syndrome (PCOS), and pregnancy may present with either primary or secondary amenorrhea.

Endocrine Determinants of Age of Menarche

The age of menarche is determined by general health and genetic, socioeconomic, and nutritional factors. The menstrual cycle involves the coordination of a series of events by the hypothalamic-pituitary-ovarian axis and is influenced by physiological, pathological, and psychological changes.

Nutrition and body weight play an important role in pubertal development. Chronic disease, malnutrition, eating disorders, and high levels of physical activity may delay menarche because of suppression

or the hypothalamic pulse generator secreting GnRH. The mechanism for this relationship is complex with the leptin, kisspeptin, neurotransmitter neuropeptide Y (NPY) pathway being the most important [3]. Leptin, secreted from white fat cells signals satiety by suppressing the activity of the central NPY, as well as stimulating appetite and eating behavior, controls GnRH activity (and therefore reproduction) as well as adrenocorticotropic hormone (ACTH) and thyroid stimulating hormone (TSH) secretion (so modifying metabolism and the response to stress). Leptin levels

Table 8B.1 Endocrine Causes of Primary Amenorrhea

Hypothalamic disorders	Constitutional delay of puberty
	Stress, exercise, weight related
	Amenorrhea, chronic illness
	Idiopathic hypogonadotrophic hypogonadism (IHH)
	Kallmann's syndrome
	Tumors (craniopharyngiomas, gliomas, germinomas, dermoid cysts)
	Cranial irradiation, head injuries (rare in young girls)
Disorders of anterior pituitary function	Pituitary adenomas
	Hypopituitarism
	Hyperprolactinaemia
	Hypothyroidism
Disorders of the ovary	Gonadal agenesis/dysgenesis, including Turner's syndrome
	Premature ovarian insufficiency
	(genetic, autoimmune, infective, radio/chemotherapy)
	Polycystic ovary syndrome (PCOS)

are low in starvation, resulting in heightened NPY activity, elevated ACTH and cortisol concentrations, and low TSH and thyroxine concentrations – as typically seen in patients with severe anorexia nervosa. As weight is regained, leptin secretion resumes, NPY activity falls, and GnRH secretion resumes, thus permitting the return of fertility as nutrition returns to normal. It is thought that leptin also plays an important role in the initiation of puberty, along with other hormones that are involved in the regulation of GnRH secretion such as kisspeptin. This may explain the key relationships between body fat and pubertal maturation observed by Frisch and Revelle [4].

Insulin has also been suggested as a modulator of the tempo of pubertal development through regulation of IGFBP-1 and sex hormone binding globulin (SHBG) [5]. In conditions of over-nutrition and obesity, the resulting increase serum concentrations of insulin, hyperinsulinemia, leads to lower levels of IGFBP-1 and reduced SHBG concentrations, thus enhancing IGF-1 and sex steroid bioavailability. Hyperandrogenism associated with PCOS may augment this situation. The converse is true in states of malnutrition, where low levels of insulin lead to increased IGFBP-1 and SHBG levels. The role of genetic factors, which may determine insulin production and obesity risk in childhood, has yet to be fully explained.

A number of other hormones interlink nutrition with reproduction, in order to prevent fertility and preserve vital bodily functions during times of famine and facilitate a return to fertility when the body is nutritionally able to cope with a pregnancy [3]. Ghrelin, secreted from the stomach, has been described as the "hunger hormone," being released during food deprivation, causing an increase in appetite and also inhibiting GnRH secretion both directly and via an increase in secretion of corticotrophin releasing hormone (CRH). Conversely, Peptide YY, from the small bowel is secreted when nutritionally replete, suppresses appetite, and stimulates GnRH pulsatility.

Endocrine Features in the Assessment of Adolescents with Primary Amenorrhea

History

Particular features of the history are important to elicit in order to evaluate a possible cause for delayed puberty and amenorrhea. Past history of intercurrent illness, weight change, and psychological stress can all influence progression through puberty. More subtle changes in dietary restriction or sporting activities can also affect hypothalamic function. Most adolescents will have a clear view of how they compare with their peer group in terms of growth and development and may even be able to identify an age when they departed from the norm. Family histories regarding the development of a sibling can also be informative.

Examination

First, a thorough assessment of auxology should be preformed with height, weight, and pubertal staging plotted against standard reference charts. Included in this assessment is the predicted height based on parent's stature. Short stature is a feature of several conditions presenting with primary amenorrhea including Turner's syndrome, hypopituitarism, and CHARGE syndrome (coloboma, heart defects, atresia choanae (also known as choanal atresia), growth retardation, genital abnormalities, and ear abnormalities). Tall stature may indicate the presence of a Y-chromosome as in Swyer syndrome, or in the older age group of delayed closure of the epiphyses as a result of estrogen deficiency. Low body weight or excessive exercise is a risk factor for hypothalamic amenorrhea with overweight being more common in PCOS. There are two components to pubertal stage. The function of estrogens is determined by Tanner staging breast development. The function of androgens is based on sexual hair development. With regard to primary amenorrhea, it is useful to contrast those with delayed or absent puberty as an estrogen-deficient subgroup from those with normal breast development as being estrogen replete, accepting there is a degree of overlap between the two.

Signs of hyperandrogenism, acne, hirsutism, and alopecia are suggestive of PCOS, although biochemical testing may be required to differentiate other causes of androgen excess. The most common is late onset congenital adrenal hyperplasia. It is important to distinguish between hyperandrogenism and virilization, which also occurs with high circulating androgen levels and causes deepening of the voice, breast atrophy, increase in muscle bulk, and cliteromegaly. A rapid onset of hirsutism suggests the possibility of an androgen-secreting tumor of the ovary or adrenal gland. Hirsutism can be graded and given a Ferriman Gallwey Score by assessing the amount of hair in

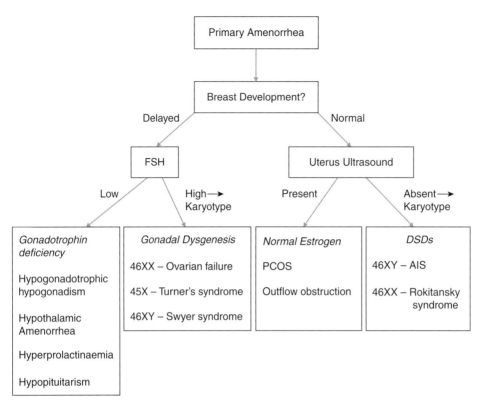

Figure 8B.1 Algorithm for the diagnosis of primary amenorrhea. Note the subgrouping based on estrogen status (breast development) and the FSH measurement. (AIS – androgen insensitivity syndrome; FSH – follicle stimulating hormone; PCOS – polycystic ovary syndrome.)

different parts of the body (e.g., upper lip, chin, breasts, abdomen, arms, legs) taking into account ethnic variations in the expression of hirsutism. Acanthosis nigricans (AN) is a sign of profound insulin resistance and is usually visible as hyperpigmented thickening of the skin folds of the axilla and neck; AN is associated with PCOS and obesity.

Vaginal examination is rarely required in the assessment of primary amenorrhea and should only be undertaken by an experienced adolescent gynecologist.

Endocrine Laboratory Investigation

The vast majority of cases of primary amenorrhea can be assessed with a simple initial profile composed of LH, FSH, prolactin, estradiol, and thyroid function [6,7]. A measurement of testosterone can be added in those with hyperandrogenism. In those with absent or delayed puberty, a measurement of FSH will distinguish between those with hypothalamic or pituitary conditions and those with gonadal dysgenesis

(Figure 8B.1). Table 8B.2 lists reference values for endocrine investigations.

A measurement of total testosterone (T) is considered adequate for general screening of hyperandrogenism. It is unnecessary to measure other androgens unless total T is >5 nmol/L (this will depend on the normal range of your local assay). Insulin may be elevated in overweight girls and suppresses the production of sex hormone binding globulin (SHBG) by the liver, resulting in a high free androgen index (FAI) in the presence of a normal total T. The measurement of SHBG is not always required in routine practice but is a useful marker for insulin resistance (IR).

A testosterone concentration > 5 nmol/L should be investigated to exclude androgen-secreting tumors of the ovary or adrenal gland, Cushing's syndrome, and late-onset congenital adrenal hyperplasia (CAH). Whereas classical salt-losing CAH often presents at birth with ambiguous genitalia, partial 21-hydroxylase deficiency may present in later life, usually in the teenage years, with signs and symptoms similar to PCOS. In such cases, T may be elevated and

Table 8B.2 Endocrine reference ranges

Note that the values will differ between laboratories depending on the assay system being used.

Follicle stimulating hormone, FSH	1–10 IU/L (early follicular)
Luteinizing hormone, LH	1–10 IU/L (early follicular)
Prolactin	<400 mIU/L
Thyroid stimulating hormone, TSH	0.5–4.0 IU/L
Thyroxine (T4)	50–150 nmol/L
Free T4	9–22 pmol/L
Tri-iodothyronine (T3)	1.5–3.5 nmol/L
Free T3	4.3–8.6 pmol/L
Thyroid binding globulin, TBG	7–17 mg/L
Testosterone (T)	0.5–3.5 nmol/L
Sex hormone binding globulin, SHBG	16–120 nmol/L
Free androgen index [(T × 100) ÷ SHBG]	<5
Dihydrotestosterone	0.3–1 nmol/L
Androstenedione	2–10 nmol/L
Dehydroepiandrosterone sulphate	3–10 µmol/L
Cortisol	
8 am	140–700 nmol/L
Midnight	0–140 nmol/L
24-hour urinary	<400 nmol/24 h
Estradiol	250–500 pmol/L
Progesterone (mid-luteal)	>25 nmol/L to indicate ovulation
17-hydroxyprogesterone	1–20 nmol/L
Inhibin B	5–200 pg/mL
Anti-Mullerian hormone (AMH)	Values should be assessed with respect to age-related nomograms. High values are often seen in adolescents and women with polycystic ovaries.

the diagnosis confirmed by an elevated serum concentration of 17-hydroxyprogesterone (17-OHP); an abnormal ACTH-stimulation test may also be helpful (250 µg ACTH will cause an elevation of 17-OHP, usually between 65 and 470 nmol/L).

The measurement of other serum androgens is only required in cases of severe hyperandrogenism, particularly those that are rapidly progressive. Dehydroepiandrosterone sulphate (DHEAS), a product of the adrenal androgen pathway, is also raised in 10 percent of women with PCOS. The measurement of androstenedione can also be useful in some situations with the benefit, in contrast to testosterone, that it is not strongly bound to SHBG.

Raised prolactin is a rare cause of primary amenorrhea; care must be taken in the interpretation of this result because this is a volatile marker of stress that can result from examination or phlebotomy. Thyroid function is included in the work-up for primary amenorrhea even though it is also a rare cause in this age group. Anti Mullerian hormone (AMH) measurements are rarely required in this age group, where AMH reflects ovarian *maturation* rather than ovarian *reserve* for which it is useful in women older than age 30 [8].

Dynamic testing of the hypothalamus using GnRH has a degree of discriminatory power to differentiate constitutional delay of puberty from hypogonadatrophic hypogonadism. Individuals with severe gonadotropin deficiency have an impaired response to GnRH stimulation; therefore, induction of puberty can be started without delay whereas those with constitutional delay may benefit from a strategy of watchful waiting.

Karyotype is only required for those presenting with raised FSH or absent uterus on ultrasound. The identification of single gene defects that cause hypogonadatrophic hypogonadism is not routinely available, although it may become so in the future [9,10]. Fragile X permutation screening is advised for ovarian insufficiency.

Endocrine Assessment with Pelvic Ultrasound

Pelvic ultrasound is an important endocrine assessment when investigating primary amenorrhea [11]. The ultrasound examination is carried out abdominally rather than vaginally; so it is essential that a sonographer experienced in transabdominal scanning performs the examination.

The size and shape of the uterus is a guide to ambient estrogen status and are generally more informative than serum estradiol concentrations that are often at the lower limit of detection [12]. In the prepubertal uterus, the cervix is the most prominent feature with a relatively small uterine body. With progression through puberty, the fundus gradually dominates both in length and later in transverse diameter. Later in puberty, the

93

endometrial thickness is a useful guide to estrogen status. It is important to note that in the absence of estrogen, the uterus may appear to be absent. Therefore, no pronouncement can be made regarding the presence of a uterus until a therapeutic trial of estrogen has been undertaken for at least 3 months [13].

The morphology of the ovary has to be interpreted with caution in individuals with primary amenorrhea. During puberty, the ovary passes through a multifollicular phase that can easily be confused with a polycystic morphology.

The morphology of the polycystic ovary has been defined as an ovary with 12 or more follicles measuring 2–9 mm in diameter and/or an increased ovarian volume (>10 cm^3) [14], although there has been subsequent data to suggest the need for >25 follicles using the latest high-definition ultrasound scanners and young women inherently have more follicles [15].

Delayed Puberty

Delayed puberty is defined as the absence of onset of puberty by greater than two standard deviations later than the average age, that is, >14 years in females. Delayed puberty may be idiopathic/familial or due to a number of general conditions resulting in undernutrition. Absence of puberty may also be due to gonadal failure (elevated gonadotrophin levels) or to impairment of gonadotrophin secretion (Table 8B.3).

In contrast to the common situation in boys, it is relatively rare for girls to present with constitutional delay of puberty. Delayed puberty due to chronic disease may respond to improved control of the associated condition. Eating disorders such as anorexia nervosa and bulimia affect 0.5 percent to 1 percent of young women in developed countries with long-term mortality rates approaching 20 percent [16]. The classic triad of presenting symptoms is weight loss in excess of 15 percent of ideal body weight, behavioral changes, and amenorrhea (secondary or primary). Adolescents with delayed puberty associated with low BMI should be carefully questioned about eating disorders, as amenorrhea may precede significant weight loss. Bulimia is associated with irregular menstruation and can occur in girls of normal weight.

Intense exercise, such as long-distance running, ballet, rowing, long-distance cycling, and gymnastics, is also associated with delayed menarche in young girls, and with amenorrhea in older women [17]. These "endurance" sports are associated with low

Table 8B.3 Causes of delayed puberty

General

- Constitutional delay of growth and puberty
- Underweight (due to severe dieting/anorexia nervosa, over-exercise or competitive sports, malabsorption such as coeliac disease or inflammatory bowel disease)
- Other chronic disease

Gonadal failure (hypergonadotrophic hypogonadism)

- o Prodromal premature ovarian failure: this is a state of ovarian insufficiency in which FSH levels are elevated and menses are irregular but not to the degree required to make a diagnosis of premature ovarian failure. It is also referred to as overt ovarian insufficiency.
- o Karyotypically normal (idiopathic) spontaneous premature ovarian failure
- o Turner's syndrome
- o Pure gonadal dysgenesis: the term "pure" here refers to the fact that the syndrome seems to have purely affected the gonad. No associated dysmorphic findings exist as are noted in Turner's syndrome, which is often referred to as gonadal dysgenesis. Pure gonadal dysgenesis can occur with either a 46 XX or a 46 XY karyotype.
- o Autoimmune oophoritis
- o 17,20-desmolase deficiency or 17-hydroxylase deficiency
- o Radiation or chemotherapy
- o Galactosaemia
- o FSH receptor mutation

Gonadotrophin deficiency

- Congenital hypogonadotrophic hypogonadism (± anosmia)
- Hypothalamic/pituitary lesions (tumors, post-radiotherapy)
- Rare inactivating mutations of genes encoding LH, FSH, or their receptors

body weight and low fat percentage. The extent to which menarche is "delayed" is related to the age at which participation in the sport begins, and to the intensity of training. Promotion of very thin women as "ideal" role models through media and fashion has contributed to an increase in dieting in adolescent girls. In addition, there are future implications for ovarian function, fertility, and sexuality and psychological support may be required at an early stage.

Gonadal failure presenting as delayed puberty requires specialist assessment and management. Unfortunately it is not uncommon for there to be long delays in both recognition and diagnosis of premature ovarian insufficiency (POI, formerly premature ovarian failure) [18], and delayed diagnosis may have serious implications for longer-term health. A karyotype is indicated to exclude Turner's syndrome (45X, or 46XX/45X mosaic) or other mosaic forms of sex chromosome anomalies. Thyroid function and thyroid and adrenal antibodies should be checked due to the association with autoimmune disease in those with a normal karyotype. The assessment of ovarian antibodies is rarely contributory because of the low sensitivity of this test. Idiopathic familial POI is well recognized and although many single gene defects have been identified, these account for only a minority of cases. For the majority of women with ovarian insufficiency, the underlying pathogenesis remains unknown.

Management of Estrogen-deficient Amenorrhea

The general principle of treatment is to replace estrogen when hypestrogenemia is demonstrated to prevent the consequences of long-term estrogen deficiency. Even short-term estrogen deficiency leads to bone loss, increasing the risk of osteoporosis. More prolonged deficiency may also increase cardiovascular risk. When a uterus is present, progestogens should also be given to avoid endometrial hyperplasia. Longitudinal studies are needed to determine the optimum replacement needed for young hyopoestrogenic women such as those with Turner's syndrome. In girls with TS, growth hormone treatment may also be used to increase stature.

Induction of Puberty

In subjects with hypogonadism, puberty should be induced as soon as delay is detected with the priority of achieving timely development in line with the peer group [19,20]. This rule applies even in Turner's syndrome where the instruction to delay the introduction of estrogen to improve final height is now considered obsolete. Low-dose estrogen is given to promote breast development; cyclical estrogen plus progestogen are then used as maintenance therapy. There is some evidence that transdermal therapy may be preferred. Ankaberg-Lindgren, Elfving, Wikland et al. [21] induced puberty in 15 girls with hypogonadotropic hypogonadism using low doses of transdermal estradiol patches attached only during the night and compared the estradiol concentrations obtained with those in healthy girls. A transdermal matrix patch of 17-beta estradiol (25 microg/24 h; Evorel, Janssen Pharmaceuticals-Cilag) can be cut into pieces corresponding to 3.1, 4.2, or 6.2 microg/24 h initially and attached to the buttock. Dose increments are made on an individual basis depending on response and

starting age. In most of the girls, breast development occurred within 3–6 months of the start of treatment.

Alternative forms of estrogen used in induction of puberty have been favored in the past, including low-dose ethinylestradiol an oral 17-beta estradiol. With the move to earlier induction of puberty, however, there has been a move away from oral preparations because the very low doses required are difficult to achieve and because more natural estradiol is thought to be favorable to synthetic estrogens such as ethinylestradiol.

PCOS in Adolescents

Polycystic ovary syndrome (PCOS) is a condition with a heterogeneous collection of signs and symptoms that gathered together form a spectrum of a disorder with a mild presentation in some, while in others there may be a severe disturbance of reproductive, endocrine, and metabolic function. The pathophysiology of the PCOS is multifactorial and polygenic, and the syndrome usually evolves during adolescence. The definition of the syndrome has been much debated, with key features including menstrual cycle disturbance, hyperandrogenism, and obesity. The joint ASRM/ESHRE consensus meeting in 2003 agreed on a refined definition of the PCOS: namely, the presence of two out of the following three criteria: (1) oligo- and/or anovulation, (2) hyperandrogenism (clinical and/or biochemical), and (3) polycystic ovaries, with the exclusion of other causes of menstrual cycle disturbance or androgen excess [22].

There is considerable heterogeneity of symptoms and signs among women with PCOS and for an individual these may change over time. The PCOS appears to be familial, and various aspects of the syndrome may be differentially inherited. Polycystic ovaries can even exist without clinical signs of the syndrome, which may then become expressed over time. A number of interlinking factors may affect expression of PCOS. For example, a gain in weight is associated with a worsening of symptoms, while weight loss may ameliorate the endocrine and metabolic profile and symptomatology. The features of obesity, hyperinsulinemia, and hyperandrogenemia, which are commonly seen in PCOS, are also known to be factors that confer an increased risk of cardiovascular disease and non-insulin-dependent diabetes mellitus (Type 2 DM). Studies indicate that women with PCOS have an increased risk for these diseases that pose long-term risks for health; this evidence has prompted debate as to the need for screening young women for polycystic ovaries.

There is no agreement concerning how to diagnose PCOS in adolescence. In fact, during the transition of girls into adulthood, several features may be in evolution or may only be transitory findings [23,24]. It has therefore been suggested that the diagnosis of PCOS should not be made until 2 years after menarche. Nonetheless, it may be useful to start treatment to address specific symptoms during the adolescent years even if the label of PCOS is not secure. Guidelines for diagnosing PCOS during adolescence have recently been proposed: namely, all elements of the Rotterdam consensus (and not just two out of three) [23]. In addition, it may be better to define hyperandrogenism as hyperandrogenemia (elevated blood androgen[s] using sensitive assays) and discount common symptoms such as acne. Oligo-amenorrhea should be present for at least 2 years and the diagnosis of polycystic ovaries by abdominal ultrasound should also include increased ovarian volume (>10 cm^3). When the diagnosis cannot be confirmed, the patients should be followed closely until adulthood, and the diagnosis should be reconsidered if the symptoms persist.

Acne is common during the adolescent years and in most subjects is a transitory phenomenon [25]. Hirsutism may be a better marker of hyperandrogenism, and some authors have reported that progressive hirsutism during the adolescent years may be an important sign of PCOS [26]. Biochemical markers, predominantly an elevated serum testosterone concentration, may also vary and do not correlate well with clinical signs [27].

Menstrual disturbance, usually oligomenorrhea and sometimes primary or secondary amenorrhea, is one of the key features of PCOS in the adult. However, in adolescence, menstrual irregularities are very common with approximately 40 percent to 85 percent having anovulatory cycles [28,29]. There is a progression toward more ovulatory cycles with increasing gynecological age, increasing from 23 percent to 35 percent during the first year after menarche to 63 percent to 65 percent by 5 years after menarche [30,31]. It has been suggested that half of adolescent girls who have oligomenorrhea or secondary amenorrhea are affected by a permanent ovulatory disorder. Various factors influence ovarian function, and fertility is adversely affected by

overweight or elevated serum concentrations of luteinizing hormone (LH).

Management of Adolescents with PCOS

Psychological, lifestyle, and dietary treatment should be the first-line approach for obese adolescent girls with PCOS. All clinical features and in particular mental disturbance are responsive to weight loss.

Combined oral contraceptive pills (OCPs) – often containing an antiandrogen – have been the mainstay for the chronic treatment of women with PCOS not seeking pregnancy. They ameliorate hyperandrogenic skin manifestations, regulate menstrual cycles, and thereby lower the risk of endometrial carcinoma, and they provide effective and safe contraception. OCPs suppress the secretion of LH and lead to a decrease in ovarian androgen production. The estrogenic fraction increases the levels of SHBG, which, in turn, results in a decrease in free T levels. The progestin in the pill can compete for 5α-reductase and the androgen receptor and thus antagonize androgen action. The OCPs also decrease adrenal androgen production, possibly due to a decrease in ACTH levels.

While almost all of the OCPs contain ethinylestradiol as the estrogenic component, progestins in the pills vary in their androgenic potential. Norethindrone, norgestrel, and levonorgestrel are known to have androgenic activity, whereas desogestrel, norgestimate, and gestodene are less androgenic. OCPs containing progestins with antiandrogenic activity rather than second- and third-generation OCPs containing progestins with varying androgenic activity appear to be an appropriate alternative in the treatment of PCOS. Among OCPs containing antiandrogenic progestins, the combination of ethinylestradiol and cyproterone acetate has been used in many studies of PCOS, whereas only a few studies of ethinylestradiol in combination with drospirenone or chlormadinone acetate are available. Recent awareness of a high thrombosis risk with oral contraceptives with antiandrogenic progestogens as well as the common side effects associated with cyproterone acetate have made this group of OCPs less popular. A similar treatment benefit can be achieved combining a third-generation OCP with low-dose antiandrogen such as spironolactone 25–50 mg daily.

Metformin, although of no benefit in older women seeking fertility, is popular in adolescence because of the coexistence of the hyperinsulinemia related to puberty and PCOS [32,33]. Metformin is also indicated in those identified with impaired glucose tolerance.

Conclusions

Estrogen deficiency in adolescence is a specialist area in terms of both investigation and management. Treatment requires a multidisciplinary approach combining experienced ultrasonography and expertise in the induction of puberty.

References

1. Marsh CA, Grimstad FW. Primary amenorrhea: diagnosis and management. *Obstetrical & Gynecological Survey* 2014; **69**: 603–12.

2. Reindollar RH, Byrd JR, McDonough PG. Delayed sexual development: a study of 252 patients. *American Journal of Obstetrics and Gynecology* 1981; **140**: 371–80.

3. Navarro VM, Tena-Sempere M. Neuroendocrine control by kisspeptins: role in metabolic regulation of fertility. *Nature Reviews Endocrinology* 2012; **8**: 40–53.

4. Frisch RE, Revelle R. Height and weight at menarche and a hypothesis of critical body weights and adolescent events. *Science* 1970; **169**: 397–99.

5. Ibanez L, Potau N, Zampolli M et al. Hyperinsulinemia and decreased insulin-like growth factor-binding protein-1 are common features in prepubertal and pubertal girls with a history of premature pubarche. *J Clin Endocrinol Metab* 1997; **82**(7): 2283–88.

6. Master-Hunter T, Heiman DL. Amenorrhea: evaluation and treatment. *American Family Physician* 2006; **73**: 1374–82.

7. Rubin K. Hypogonadism in adolescent females: new insights and rationale supporting the use of physiologic regimens to induce puberty. *Pediatric Endocrinology Reviews: PER* 2005; **2**: 645–52.

8. Hagen CP, Mouritsen A, Mieritz MG et al. Circulating AMH reflects ovarian morphology by magnetic resonance imaging and 3D ultrasound in 121 healthy girls. *The Journal of Clinical Endocrinology and Metabolism* 2015; **100**: 880–90.

9. Bry-Gauillard H, Trabado S, Bouligand J et al. Congenital hypogonadotropic hypogonadism in females: clinical spectrum, evaluation and genetics. *Annales d'endocrinologie.* 2010; **71**: 158–62.

10. Layman LC. The genetic basis of female reproductive disorders: etiology and clinical testing. *Molecular and Cellular Endocrinology* 2013; **370**: 138–48.

11. Paltiel HJ, Phelps A. US of the pediatric female pelvis. *Radiology* 2014; **270**: 644–57.

12. Bumbuliene Z, Klimasenko J, Sragyte D et al. Uterine size and ovarian size in adolescents with functional hypothalamic amenorrhea. *Archives of Disease in Childhood* 2015; **100**: 948–51.

13. Michala L, Aslam N, Conway GS et al. The clandestine uterus: or how the uterus escapes detection prior to puberty. *BJOG: An International Journal of Obstetrics and Gynecology* 2010; **117**: 212–15.

14. Balen A, Laven J, Tan S et al. Ultrasound assessment of the polycystic ovary: international consensus definitions. *Hum. Rep. Update* 2003; **9**(6): 505–14.

15. Dewailly D, Lujan ME, Carmina E et al. Definition and significance of polycystic ovarian morphology: a task force report from the Androgen Excess And Polycystic Ovary Syndrome Society. *Hum Reprod Update* 2014; **20**: 334–52.

16. Tamburrino MB, McGinnis RA Anorexia nervosa. A review. *Panminerva Med Dec* 2002; **44**(4): 301–11.

17. Joy E, De Souza MJ, Nattiv A et al. Female athlete triad coalition consensus statement on treatment and return to play of the female athlete triad. *Current Sports Medicine Reports* 2014; **13**: 219–32.

18. Alzubaidi NH, Chapin HL, Vanderhoof VH et al. Meeting the needs of young women with secondary amenorrhea and spontaneous premature ovarian failure. *Obstet Gynecol* 2002; **99**(5 Pt 1): 720–25.

19. Delemarre EM, Felius B, Delemarre-van de Waal HA. Inducing puberty. *European Journal of Endocrinology/European Federation of Endocrine Societies* 2008; **159** Suppl 1: S9–15.

20. MacGillivray MH. Induction of puberty in hypogonadal children. *Journal of Pediatric Endocrinology & Metabolism : JPEM* 2004; **17** Suppl 4: 1277–87.

21. Ankarberg-Lindgren C, Elfving M, Wikland KA et al. Nocturnal application of transdermal estradiol patches produces levels of estradiol that mimic those seen at the onset of spontaneous puberty in girls. *J Clin Endocrinol Metab* (2001); **86**(7): 3039–44.

22. Rotterdam ESHRE/ASRM-Sponsored PCOS Consensus Workshop Group. Revised 2003 consensus on diagnostic criteria and long-term health risks related to polycystic ovary syndrome (PCOS). *Hum Reprod* 2014; **19**: 41–47.

23. Carmina E, Oberfield SE, Lobo RA. The diagnosis of polycystic ovary syndrome in adolescents. *Am J Obstet Gynecol* 2010; **203**: 201–5.

24. Fauser BCJM, Tarlatzis BC, Rerbar RW et al. Consensus on women's health aspects of polycystic ovary syndrome (PCOS): the Amsterdam ESHRE/ASRM-Sponsored 3rd PCOS Consensus Workshop Group. *Human Reproduction* 2012; **27**: 14–24 and *Fertility & Sterility* 2012; **97**: 28–38.

25. Olutunmbi Y, Paley K, English JC, III. Adolescent female acne: etiology and management. *J Pediatr Adolesc Gynecol* 2008; **21**: 171–76.

26. Jeffrey CR, Coffler MS. Polycystic ovary syndrome: early detection in the adolescent. *Clin Obstet Gynecol* 2007; **50**: 178–87.

27. Blank SK, Helm KD, McCartney CR et al. Polycystic ovary syndrome in adolescence. *Ann N Y Acad Sci* 2001; **1135**: 76–84.

28. Apter D. Endocrine and metabolic abnormalities in adolescents with a PCOS-like condition: consequences for adult reproduction. *Trends Endocrinol Metab* 1998; **9**: 58–61.

29. Metcalf MG, Skidmore DS, Lowry GF et al. Incidence of ovulation in the years after the menarche. *J Endocrinol* 1983; **97**: 213–19.

30. Venturoli S, Porcu E, Fabbri F et al. Menstrual irregularities in adolescents: hormonal pattern and ovarian morphology. *Horm Res* 1986; **24**: 269–79.

31. Wiksten-Almstromer M, Hirschberg AL, Hagenfeldt K. Prospective follow-up of menstrual disorders in adolescence and prognostic factors. *Acta Obstet Gynecol Scand* 2008; **87**: 1162–68.

32. De Leo V, Musacchio MC, Morgante G et al. Metformin treatment is effective in obese teenage girls with PCOS. *Human Reproduction* (Oxford, England). 2006; **21**: 2252–56.

33. Hoeger K, Davidson K, Kochman L et al. The impact of metformin, oral contraceptives, and lifestyle modification on polycystic ovary syndrome in obese adolescent women in two randomized, placebo-controlled clinical trials. *The Journal of Clinical Endocrinology and Metabolism* 2008; **93**: 4299–306.

Primary Amenorrhea in Pediatric and Adolescent Gynecology practice
Mayer-Rokitansky-Kuster-Hauser Syndrome

Ephia Yasmin and Gail Busby

Introduction

Mayer-Rokitansky-Kuster-Hauser (MRKH) syndrome is a condition characterized by the absence of a functioning uterus, a short or absent vagina, normal secondary sexual characteristics, normal ovarian function, and a female karyotype [1]. The syndrome is one of the commonest disorders of sex development (DSD) [2] and accounts for just under 3 percent of Müllerian abnormalities [3]. Following the first descriptions by Mayer (1829) and Rokitansky (1838), Kuster (1910) reviewed cases with absent uteri from the literature in 1910. Hauser added his name to this syndrome calling it Mayer-Rokitansky-Kuster-Hauser in 1961 [4]. The incidence of this condition has been quoted to be 1 in 4, 500 to 5, 000 female births [1].

The MRKH syndrome predominantly exists in three types (Table 8C.1). Renal, skeletal, hearing, or rarely cardiac congenital anomalies are associated with MRKH [6]. Typical MRKH exists with no other genital malformation. Atypical MRKH is associated with malformations in the renal system and Müllerian duct aplasia, renal aplasia, and cervicothoracic somite dysplasia or MURCS when associated with renal and skeletal abnormalities [5]. In a study of 283 women with MRKH, Oppelt et al. [7] found the following

Table 8C.1 Types of MRKH

MRKH Syndrome	Associated Malformations
Typical	Tubes, ovaries, and renal system normal
Atypical	Malformations of the ovary or renal system
MURCS	Malformations in the skeleton and/or heart; muscular weakness, renal malformations

MURCS = Müllerian aplasia, renal aplasia, and cervicothoracic somite dysplasia

frequencies: typical MRKH 54.9 percent, atypical MRKH 26 percent, and MURCS 13.4 percent.

Embryology of the Female Reproductive System

A brief synopsis of the embryological development of the reproductive structures and the renal system is presented to understand MRKH syndrome. In females, the Müllerian (paramesonephric) ducts arise from the mesoderm lateral to the mesonephric ducts at the 7th week of gestation (Figure 8C.1). Normal development of the Müllerian system depends on the completion of three phases: organogenesis, fusion, and septal resorption. The Müllerian ducts grow caudally, lateral to the urogenital ridges. They subsequently fuse to form a confluence that is a precursor to the upper two-thirds of the vagina, the cervix, the body of the uterus, and the Fallopian tubes. The unfused cranial ends of the Müllerian ducts form the Fallopian tubes, which open into the coelomic cavity (Figure 8C.1). The renal system develops in three stages: pronephros, mesonephros, and metanephros. The paired pronephros involute by the 5th week. The mesonephros forms in the 4th week. The Wolffian (mesonephric) ducts drain the mesonephros into the cloaca ventrally and nephrogenic cords laterally. The mesonephros and Wolffian ducts regress by the 3rd month and the metanephros eventually becomes the kidney. Arrested development and failed fusion of the Müllerian ducts lead to MRKH syndrome. Due to the close association of the Müllerian and caudal parts of the mesonephric duct, renal agenesis or ectopia can be associated with MRKH. Gonadal differentiation takes place at 7 weeks of fetal life. The primitive germ cells migrate to the genital ridge from the primitive yolk sac leading to the formation of the ovaries. Due to a separate embryological origin of the ovaries, they are spared in MRKH syndrome [1].

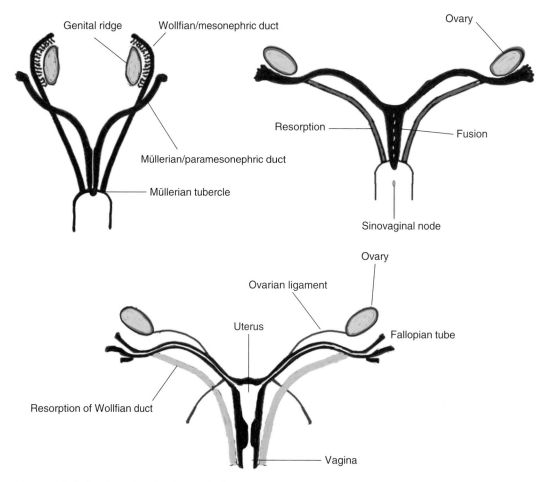

Figure 8C.1 Embryology of the female reproductive system

There are several classifications of Müllerian anomalies. According to the American Fertility Society classification (1988), MRKH falls into the first class of anomalies. In the CONUTA classification, MRKH is incorporated into class U5 of anomalies [9]. The U5 group of anomalies is further subdivided depending on the presence or absence of a functional cavity within a rudimentary uterus. Class U5a is characterized by the presence of a bi- or uni-lateral functional horn and class U5b by the presence of uterine tissue without a functional cavity and complete absence of any uterine tissue.

Diagnosis of MRKH Syndrome

The MRKH syndrome is usually identified when the individual presents with primary amenorrhea. Patients may report to primary care at age 13 or 14;

however, due to the presence of normal secondary sexual characteristics, investigations or referral to secondary care may not take place until age 16. Some patients may present with unsuccessful attempts at coitus. Cyclical recurrent lower abdominal pain may result from endometrial proliferation within uterine buds (anlagan) if they contain active endometrium or from endometriosis, adenomyosis and myomas, which have been described in 6-10 percent of patients with MRKH syndrome [10]. History will reveal pubarche and thelarche at the usual time. In a study by Michala et al. [11], 53 percent of women with MRKH were found to have urinary symptoms. Therefore, a history of urinary function should be taken and any recurrent urinary problems need to be monitored.

Examination reveals normal female external genitalia. A small dimple or a short vagina may be seen.

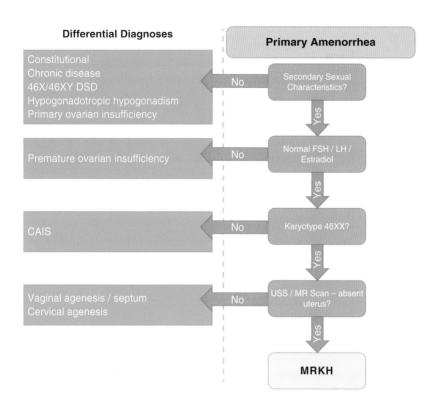

Differential Diagnoses

Figure 8C.2 Flowchart for diagnosis of MRKH

MRI examination should ideally be performed to evaluate the pelvis and the urinary system. Ultrasound examination may be inconclusive depending on the experience of the operator. Although imaging usually reports an absent uterus, some rudimentary uterine buds are present in about 90 percent of MRKH patients. Hall-Craggs and coauthors [15] detected single or bipartite rudimentary uteri, which are often bilateral, in 92 percent of women with MRKH (Figure 8C.3). Ectopic ovaries were found either bilaterally or unilaterally. The ectopic ovaries were positioned in the pelvis either antero-laterally or far laterally and high in the pelvis just below the pelvic brim. Information on location of the ovaries is important when the patients wish to undergo fertility treatment. The route of oocyte retrieval will depend on the location of the ovaries.

An examination under anesthesia is rarely required to make a diagnosis of MRKH. An ultrasound examination of the abdomen and pelvis or an MRI will usually provide adequate information [12].

Women with MRKH usually have a 46XX karyotype, normal gonadotrophins, and normal serum estrogen and testosterone levels [1]. Some patients with MRKH may also have clinical and biochemical hyperandrogenism along with polycystic ovary morphology [16]. A very low concentration of gonadotrophins with low estrogen suggests hypogonadotrophic hypogonadism (HH), and elevated gonadotrophins with low estradiol points toward premature ovarian insufficiency (POI) as the cause of primary amenorrhea. Both these conditions may inhibit development of the uterus leading to the suggestion of absent uterus on imaging studies and an incorrect diagnosis of MRKH syndrome. Michala and colleagues demonstrated the difficulty of diagnosing the absence of uteri before puberty and recommended that the diagnosis of an absent uterus should only be made after puberty or after estrogen supplementation in HH and POI [14]. A state of hypoestrogenism (HH, POI) may sometimes be confused with

MRKH due to the presence of a small prepubertal uterus. Low or elevated gonadotrophins will help in diagnosis and estrogen supplementation will usually lead to the development of the uterus in POI and HH. Figure 8C.2 presents a flow chart showing the algorithm for diagnosis of MRKH.

A study by Rall et al. [16] also revealed uterine rudiments showing a duct-like structure or small cavity, few of which contained endometrium. All rudiments contained an intact myometrial layer. Tubal epithelium and stroma were found in three rudimentary uteri. No significant differences were observed with regard to estrogen receptor (ER) or progesterone receptor (PR) expression in endometrium or myometrium.

Due to association of renal abnormalities with Müllerian anomalies, the assessment of the renal tract forms part of the routine investigation of patients presenting with Müllerian anomalies. In the largest series reporting the incidence of renal anomalies in patients with Müllerian duct anomalies (MDAs), unilateral renal agenesis has been reported in around 30 percent of patients. Other abnormalities are ectopic kidneys and ureters, duplex kidneys and ureters, and horseshoe kidney [17].

Genetics of MRKH Syndrome

The question that parents of girls with MRKH and MRKH patients often ask is the cause of the anomaly and whether the syndrome is genetically inherited. There is no clear evidence about whether MRKH is genetic, environmental, or both. The syndrome was initially considered to be a sporadic anomaly, but more recent literature supports a genetic link although no single gene defect has been identified [1]. The genetic mutations that have been investigated due to their roles in the development and differentiation of the female reproductive and urinary tract are listed in Table 8C.2.

It is safe to say that Müllerian anomalies display multifactorial rather than single gene inheritance. In familial cases, the syndrome appears to be transmitted as an autosomal dominant trait with incomplete penetrance and variable expressivity, which suggests the involvement of either mutations in a major developmental gene or a limited chromosomal imbalance [18,19]. Women with MRKH have not been shown to have increased abnormalities in offsprings. In a study of 58 women with MRKH undergoing infertility treatment with gestational surrogates, none of the 17 female infants born exhibited MRKH [20]. However, women with MRKH and other associated anomalies (renal, skeletal) may be more likely to have children with abnormalities [21].

Table 8C.2 Genetics and MRKH

Gene	Chromosome	Cytogenetic band
PAX2	10	10q24
WT1	11	11p13
HOXA 7	7	7p15.2
HOXA13	7	7p15.2
WNT4	1	1p36.23–p35.1

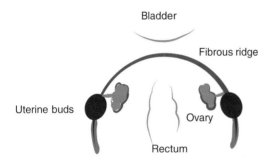

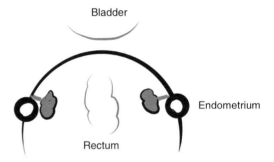

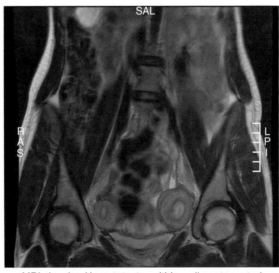

MRI showing Hematometra within rudimentary uteri

Figure 8C.3 Variations in Müllerian duct development in MRKH

In the light of this evidence or lack thereof, patients with MRKH should be counseled that their genetic offspring are likely to exhibit normal Müllerian anatomy at birth. No single gene defects have been identified to allow for preimplantation genetic diagnosis of the condition. Women in whom MRKH coincides with musculoskeletal, vertebral, or cardiac conditions may be more likely to pass their disorders to their children but this assumption requires more studies to establish this link.

Management of MRKH Syndrome

The management of MRKH syndrome includes three main aspects of care: neovagina creation, fertility issues, and psychological support. To adequately address all of these issues, the care of these patients should be delivered by a multidisciplinary team experienced in the management of these cases. The team should include a gynecologist, psychologist, nurse specialist, fertility specialist, and radiologist.

Psychological Support in MRKH

Beyond the physical issue of vaginal agenesis and infertility, there are social and psychological issues that affect women with MRKH [22]. Studies have demonstrated that women experience negative emotions on diagnosis. Patients report feelings of compromised femininity and threat to identifying as a woman [23,24]. The inability to carry a pregnancy is a significant source of distress [25]. The importance of general adjustment and psychological well-being has been recognized as being an important predictor of positive sexual functioning; therefore, psychological support should precede any medical therapies such as creation of neovagina. Moreover, psychological support should also aim to assist and empower the patient to make decisions about their sexuality, fertility, nature and timing of any medical assistance.

Creation of Neovagina

A few patients may be sexually active at presentation, having had natural dilation of the vaginal dimple due to repeated coitus. These patients require no further treatment for neovagina, unless they cease sexual activity, in which case dilation will be necessary to maintain the vaginal length. Dilation procedures for vaginal hypoplasia or agenesis in nonsexually experienced women include nonsurgical dilation therapy and surgical vaginoplasty [26].

Vaginal Dilation Therapy

In 1938, Frank described the use of Pyrex® tubes of gradually increasing sizes (0.8, 1.5, and 2.0 cm in diameter) to stretch the mucous membrane inward into the introital region. For almost 40 years, this technique was only infrequently used. The downsides to this technique were fatigue of manual effort and the inability to engage in any other activities. To avoid the need to manually stretch and elongate the vaginal dimple, Ingram modified the technique in 1981 by inserting dilators into the saddle of a bicycle stool on which patients could sit astride to create pressure [28]. The seat was later modified by Lee [27] and Lankford and Haefner [29]. However these modifications involved bigger contraptions as opposed to the dilators that could be contained in a small box or case and therefore were more portable.

The ACOG [30] in 2002 recommended nonsurgical vaginal dilation as the first-choice treatment, because it is a patient-driven technique that is easy to perform, cost–effective, and safe. Successful neovaginal creation by dilation obviates the need for major surgery in most patients. It is expected that about 85 percent of women will achieve a functional vagina without a surgical approach [31,32]. The same group quoted a 94.9 percent success with creation of neovagina in patients who completed the vaginal dilation program [31]. This study was criticized for taking an arbitrary vaginal length of 6 cm as the outcome measure and not elaborating on how sexual satisfaction was evaluated [22]. Reasons for failure of vaginal self-dilation require further research. Failed vaginal dilation therapy may further jeopardize surgical vaginoplasty as most of these procedures require ongoing vaginal dilation.

Surgical Vaginoplasty

In the UK, surgical vaginoplasty is offered if vaginal dilation therapy fails. In other European countries, this is used as a first line for neovagina creation [34]. Surgical vaginoplasty began with creation of a pouch between the rectum and bladder. This was followed by split thickness skin grafts taken from the thigh or buttock that were inserted over the mold, after dissection of the space between the rectum and bladder. There were proponents of various types of skin grafts (pudendal thigh flaps, free flap graft from the vulvoperineal fasciocutaneous flaps). The drawbacks of most of these techniques were scars and keloid formation, lack of vaginal lubrication, hair regrowth in the Neovagina, and vaginal stenosis. It is rarely performed in the UK for MRKH [36].

Vecchietti Procedure

In 1965, Vecchietti proposed a device that used an upward traction on the vaginal dimple exerted by an acrylic olive in the vagina. The upward traction on the olive was created with the help of a device attached to the anterior abdominal wall into which the threads leading from the olive were connected. These threads were tightened daily for a week leading to the rapid creation of a neovaginal space [37]. This procedure was initially performed via laparotomy. The laparoscopic adaptation proposed in 1992 obviated the need for a large incision, thus improving healing and recovery [38]. The neovaginal epithelium is found to be macroscopically similar to normal vaginal mucosa. The complication rate including bladder and rectal wall injury was reported to be low [34]. A drawback for this procedure is its invasive nature and the pain resulting from the sustained traction that necessitates hospital stay for the duration of traction. Effective analgesia is needed during that time [26]. Vault prolapses have been reported after neovagina creation although not common [39]. This has been successfully treated by sacrospinous ligament suspension.

Davydov's Procedure

Davydov developed a three-stage operation involving dissection of the rectovesical space with abdominal mobilization of the peritoneum, attachment of the peritoneum to the created introitus, and finally closure of the neovaginal vault with purse-string suture [40]. The claimed advantage of this technique by the authors is the lack of granulation tissue and scar formation. The procedure was modified to a laparoscopic approach, having the advantages of reduced blood loss and postoperative pain in addition to shorter hospital stay, faster recovery, and better cosmetic outcome [41].

Bowel Vaginoplasty

Use of ileal or sigmoid caecum loop for creation of neovagina has been described since the early 1900s. A laparoscopic approach has been carried out since 1996 [42], but the procedure is still most frequently performed through a laparotomy. The main advantages of this operation are said to be the lack of shrinkage with no requirement for long-term vaginal dilation and the natural lubrication provided by the mucous production that obviates the need for artificial lubricants and decreases the risk of dyspareunia [42]. These procedures are associated with greater morbidity than nonsurgical and laparoscopic approaches [2] and are seldom required in MRKH syndrome. Furthermore, many patients describe chronic unpleasant discharge as a consequence of mucosal secretions, which has led to requests for removal of the transposed bowel.

Creatsas Modification of Williams Vaginoplasty

Creatsas modified the Williams vaginoplasty by making a U-shaped incision in the vulva, starting at 4 cm lateral to the external urethral meatus and the medial side of the labia majora, extending down to the perineum and up the other side of the vulva. A layer of sutures is then placed on the inner skin margins to create a pouch. The perineal muscles and subcutaneous tissue are mobilized and approximated, before the external skin is closed. With this technique, vaginal dilation is not necessary and coitus can be commenced once the surgical wounds have healed. Of 200 patients undergoing this procedure, 95.5 percent have a vagina of length 10–12 cm and width 5 cm; 94.5 percent of patients reported a satisfactory quality of sexual life post-procedure. This last assessment, however, was not performed with a validated questionnaire [43].

Other Techniques of Neovagina

Various other authors have reported on the use of artificial or biological materials, including buccal mucosa, artificial dermis (atelocollagen sponge), basic fibroblast growth factor to accelerate epithelization, oxidized cellulose, and autologous in vitro–cultured vaginal tissue [44].

In summary, creation of neovagina can usually be achieved with patient-driven dilation with psychological support and supervision from a trained nurse specialist. Where vaginal self-dilation fails to achieve vaginal capacity for penetrative sex, laparoscopic Vecchietti procedure can be offered with subsequent self-dilation to maintain patency. Very rarely the Davydov procedure may need to be used (Figure 8C.4).

Measuring Success with Nonsurgical and Surgical Neovagina

It is difficult to quantify anatomic and functional success of vaginal dilation. Reference values for

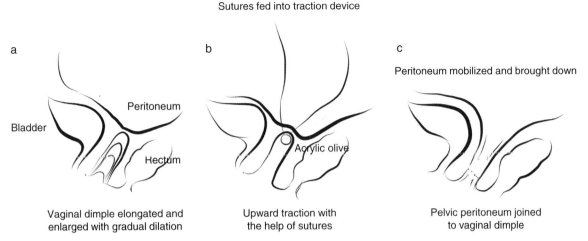

Sutures fed into traction device

a

b

c

Peritoneum mobilized and brought down

Peritoneum

Bladder

Rectum

Acrylic olive

Vaginal dimple elongated and
enlarged with gradual dilation

Upward traction with
the help of sutures

Pelvic peritoneum joined
to vaginal dimple

Figure 8C.4 Procedures for neovagina in MRKH
a. Vaginal dilation, b. Vecchietti procedure, c. Davydov procedure

normal vaginal length have been described as 7–13 cm (mean 9.25 + 1.56 cm) [45]. Few studies have suggested 6 cm of vaginal length to be optimal. However, although an objective physical examination might reveal a suboptimal anatomic result, this has not been found to correlate with the patient's interpretation of successful outcome. The review by Bean [47] revealed that surgical or nonsurgical creation of a neovagina alone does not ensure a successful psychological outcome. The review emphasizes the importance of psychological support and the language of counseling on the part of clinicians as they influence a patient's experience significantly.

Liao and coauthors [22] assessed 58 women with MRKH syndrome. Compared with normative data, participants were found to have overall good physical health but poorer mental health. Anxiety levels were found to be higher, especially for women who had undergone vaginal treatment. Sexual wellness and function scores were observed to be poor. Vaginal length was found to have a positive correlation with overall sexual satisfaction although not related to overall quality of life. Morcel, Lavoué, Jaffre, Paniel, and Rouzier [46] reported similar functional sexual outcomes after nonsurgical and surgical vaginoplasty.

Vaginal dilation therapy should only be started once psychological evaluation and support are in place. Psychological support encompasses acceptance of the diagnosis, coping strategies, disclosure strategies, and improvement off self-esteem and quality of life. Optimal time to start therapy is when the patient wishes to do so [2].

Fertility in MRKH Syndrome

The lack of innate reproductive potential has been one of the most emotionally detrimental aspects of MRKH syndrome and is recognized as one of the most important concerns in women with MRKH [25]. Fertility counseling is a key feature of MRKH management. Motherhood options for the MRKH syndrome patient have been adoption and gestational surrogacy [48]. For women with MRKH who wish to start a family, a referral to the fertility specialist is warranted. Host surrogacy involves carrying out controlled ovarian stimulation and IVF in the intended parent and preparation of the surrogate to receive a fresh or frozen embryo. Surrogacy laws differ in various countries. In the UK, surrogacy is legal (www.hfea.gov.uk/501.html). Nonprofit organizations such as Surrogacy UK assist intended parents in meeting a potential surrogate. Relatives, family members, and friends can also choose to be host surrogates. Commercial surrogacy exists overseas, but in the UK it should be altruistic. The state funding of surrogacy varies around the UK. The benefits of surrogacy are the reliability of the IVF process especially when maternal age is younger than age 35 [49]. The risks are those of ovarian hyperstimulation syndrome and access to ovaries for egg collection. As the ovaries are generally situated higher in MRKH syndrome [15], access to them transvaginally may be a challenge. However, abdominal or laparoscopic egg collections are alternatives to vaginal oocyte retrievals [49].

Uterine Transplant

With the first live birth following uterine transplant in an MRKH syndrome patient [50], this procedure has gained a lot of attention. The Brannstrom group has carried out nine uterine transplants with four live births and one ongoing pregnancy as of October 2015. Two of the transplants were removed, one due to uterine artery thrombosis and the other to infection. Mild rejection episodes occurred in five out of seven patients. Two patients had preeclampsia during pregnancy. The Brannstom group used live donors. The intention is to remove the allografts once childbearing is complete, thereby restricting the time the patients are on immunosuppressants [50]. One patient is now pregnant for the second time. Cadaveric uterine donors are also a possibility. The concern with cadaveric uteri is ischemia, which may decrease graft function.

There are several ethical concerns about uterine transplants [52]. The procedure is non-vital and involves two high-risk procedures if a live donor is used. The surgical risk to the donor is significant and is alleviated with the use of deceased donors. The ethics of paid organ donation also arises once this procedure comes into common practice. On the other hand, in some countries, such as Sweden, surrogacy is illegal. The Swedish group has emphasized that uterine transplant needs to be performed only in the research setting and more data need to be gathered with the help of international registries.

Conclusion

Mayer-Rokitansky-Kuster-Hauser syndrome is a rare condition but forms the majority of DSDs in specialist clinics. The possibility of MRKH should be considered in the event of the presentation of primary amenorrhea in the presence of normal secondary sexual characteristics in an adolescent female. The diagnosis is made by history, clinical examination, karyotyping, gonadotrophin and estradiol levels, and imaging of the pelvis. As renal or vertebral anomalies can coexist, these must be assessed and investigated if necessary. No single gene disorder has been linked to MRKH. The management of MRKH syndrome must recognize that it carries a huge psychological burden. Management needs to be multidisciplinary. Vaginal dilation techniques have good anatomical outcome but functional outcomes need more research. Reporting of outcome measures needs to be standardized to compare results in a meaningful way. Fertility is one of the main concerns for the individual and in-depth fertility counseling is required to assist the patient in the decision-making process. Uterine transplantation is still in the research phase, but it holds promise to become a mainstream operation in the future.

References

1. Pizzo A, Laganà AS, Sturlese E, Retto G, Retto A, De Dominici R, Puzzolo D. Mayer-Rokitansky-Kuster-Hauser syndrome: embryology, genetics and clinical and surgical treatment. *ISRN Obstet Gynecol* 2013; 628717.

2. Nakhal RS, Creighton SM. Management of vaginal agenesis. *J Pediatr Adolesc Gynecol* 2012; **25**(6): 352–57.

3. Grimbizis GF, Camus M, Tarlatzis BC, Bontis JN, Devroey P. Clinical implications of uterine malformations and hysteroscopic treatment results. *Hum Reprod Update* 2001; 7(2): 161–74.

4. Hauser GA, Keller M, Koller T, Wenner R. The Rokitansky-Kuester-syndrome. Uterus bipartitus solidus rudimentarius cum vagina solida. *Gynecologia* 1961; **151**: 111–12.

5. Schmid-Tannwald I, Hauser GA Atypical forms of the Mayer–Rokitansky–Kuester syndrome. *Geburtshilfe Frauenheilkd* 1977; **37**: 386–92.

6. Duncan PA, Shapiro LR, Stangel JJ, Klein RM and Addonizio JC The MURCS association: Müllerian duct aplasia, renal aplasia, and cervicothoracic somite dysplasia. *J Pediatr* 1979; **95**: 399–402.

7. Oppelt PG, Lermann J, Strick R, Dittrich R, Strissel P, Rettig I et al. Malformations in a cohort of 284 women with Mayer-Rokitansky-Kuster-Hauser syndrome (MRKH). *Reprod Biol Endocrinol* 2012; **20** (10): 57.

8. The American Fertility Society. Classifications of adnexal adhesions, distal tubal occlusion, tubal occlusion secondary to tubal ligation, tubal pregnancies, müllerian anomalies and intrauterine adhesions. *Fertil Steril* 1988; **49**(6): 944–55.

9. Grimbizis GF, Gordts S, Di Spiezio Sardo A, Brucker S, De Angelis C, Gergolet M et al. The ESHRE-ESGE consensus on the classification of female genital tract congenital anomalies. *Gynecol Surg* 2013; **10**(3): 199–212.

10. Marsh CA, Will MA, Smorgick N, Quint EH, Hussain H, Smith YR. Uterine remnants and pelvic pain in females with Mayer-Rokitansky-Kuster-Hauser syndrome. *J Pediatr Adolesc Gynecol* 2013; **26**(3): 199–202.

11. Michala L, Strawbridge L, Bikoo M, Cutner AS, Creighton SM. Lower urinary tract symptoms in

women with vaginal agenesis. *Int Urogynecol J* 2013; **24** (3): 425–29.

12. Rousset P, Raudrant D, Peyron N, Buy JN, Valette PJ, Hoeffel C. Ultrasonography and MRI features of the Mayer-Rokitansky-Kuster-Hauser syndrome. *Clin Radiol* 2013; **68**(9): 945–52.

13. Rall K, Conzelmann G, Schäffeler N, Henes M, Wallwiener D, Möhrle M, Brucker SY. Acne and PCOS are less frequent in women with Mayer-Rokitansky-Kuster-Hauser syndrome despite a high rate of hyperandrogenemia: a cross-sectional study. *Reprod Biol Endocrinol* 2014; **12**: 23.

14. Michala L, Aslam N, Conway GS, Creighton SM. The clandestine uterus: or how the uterus escapes detection prior to puberty. *BJOG.* 2010; **117**(2): 212–25.

15. Hall-Craggs MA, Williams CE, Pattison SH, Kirkham AP, Creighton SM. Mayer-Rokitansky-Kuster-Hauser syndrome: diagnosis with MR imaging. *Radiology.* 2013; **269**(3): 787–92.

16. Rall K, Barresi G, Wallwiener D, Brucker SY, Staebler A. Uterine rudiments in patients with Mayer-Rokitansky-Kuster-Hauser syndrome consist of typical uterine tissue types with predominantly basalis-like endometrium. *Fertil Steril* 2013; **99**(5): 1392–99.

17. Rall K, Eisenbeis S, Henninger V, Henes M, Wallwiener D, Bonin M, Brucker S. Typical and atypical associated findings in a group of 346 patients with Mayer-Rokitansky-Kuester-Hauser syndrome. *J Pediatr Adolesc Gynecol* 2015; **28**(5): 362–68.

18. Layman LC. The genetic basis of female reproductive disorders: etiology and clinical testing. *Mol Cell Endocrinol* 2013; **370**(1–2): 138–48.

19. Morcel K, Camborieux L. Programme de Recherches sur les Aplasies Mul[é]riennes, Guerrier D. Mayer-Rokitansky-Kuster-Hauser (MRKH) syndrome. *Orphanet J Rare Dis* 2007; **2**: 13.

20. Petrozza JC, Gray MR, Davis AJ, Reindollar RH. Congenital absence of the uterus and vagina is not commonly transmitted as a dominant genetic trait: outcomes of surrogate pregnancies. *Fertil Steri.* 1997; **67**(2): 387–89.

21. Philibert P, Biason-Lauber A, Rouzier R, Pienkowski C, Paris F, Konrad D et al. Identification and functional analysis of a new WNT4 gene mutation among 28 adolescent girls with primary amenorrhea and Müllerian duct abnormalities: a French collaborative study. *J Clin Endocrinol Metab.* 2008; **93** (3): 895–900.

22. Liao LM, Conway GS, Ismail-Pratt I, Bikoo M, Creighton SM. Emotional and sexual wellness and quality of life in women with Rokitansky syndrome. *Am J Obstet Gynecol* 2011; **205**(2): 117.e1–6.

23. Vates TS, Fleming P, Leleszi JP, Barthold JS, González R, Perlmutter AD. Functional, social and psychosexual adjustment after vaginal reconstruction. *J Uro.* 1999; **162**(1): 182–87.

24. Giannesi A, Marchiole P, Benchaib M, Chevret-Measson M, Mathevet P, Dargent D. Sexuality after laparoscopic Davydov in patients affected by congenital complete vaginal agenesis associated with uterine agenesis or hypoplasia. *Hum Reprod.* 2005; **20**(10): 2954–57.

25. Kimberley N, Hutson JM, Southwell BR, Grover SR. Well-being and sexual function outcomes in women with vaginal agenesis. *Fertil Steril* 2011; **95**(1): 238–41.

26. Deans R, Berra M, Creighton SM. Management of vaginal hypoplasia in disorders of sexual development: surgical and non-surgical options. *Sex Dev* 2010; **4**(4–5): 292–99.

27. Lee MH. Non-surgical treatment of vaginal agenesis using a simplified version of Ingram's method. *Yonsei Med J* 2006; **47**(6): 892–95.

28. Ingram JM. The bicycle seat stool in the treatment of vaginal agenesis and stenosis: a preliminary report. *Am J Obstet Gynecol* 1981; **140**(8): 867–73.

29. Lankford JA, Haefner HK. Modification of the Ingram bicycle seat stool for the treatment of vaginal agenesis and stenosis. *Int J Gynaecol Obstet* 2008; **102**(3): 301–3.

30. American College of Obstetrics and Gynecology. Committee on Adolescent Health Care. ACOG committee opinion. Number 274. Nonsurgical diagnosis and management of vaginal agenesis. *Int J Gynaecol Obstet* 2002; **79**(2): 167–70.

31. Edmonds DK, Rose GL, Lipton MG, Quek J. Mayer-Rokitansky-Kuster-Hauser syndrome: a review of 245 consecutive cases managed by a multidisciplinary approach with vaginal dilators. *Fertil Steril* 2012; **97**(3): 686–90.

32. Bach F, Glanville JM, Balen AH. An observational study of women with müllerian agenesis and their need for vaginal dilator therapy. *Fertil Steril* 2011; **96**(2): 483–86.

33. Creighton S, Crouch N, Deans R, Cutner A, Michala L, Barnett M et al. Nonsurgical dilation for vaginal agenesis is promising, but better research is needed. *Fertil Steril* 2012; **97**(6).

34. Callens N, De Cuypere G, De Sutter P, Monstrey S, Weyers S, Hoebeke P, Cools M. An update on surgical and non-surgical treatments for vaginal hypoplasia. *Hum Reprod Update* 2014; **20**(5): 775–801.

35. McIndoe A. The treatment of congenital absence and obliterative conditions of the vagina. *Br J Plast Surg* 1950; **2**(4): 254–67.

36. Ismail-Pratt IS, Bikoo M, Liao LM, Conway GS, Creighton SM. Normalization of the vagina by dilator

treatment alone in complete androgen insensitivity syndrome and Mayer-Rokitansky-Kuster-Hauser syndrome. *Hum Reprod* 2007; **22**(7): 2020–24.

37. Vecchietti G. Creation of an artificial vagina in Rokitansky-Kuster-Hauser syndrome. *Attual Ostet Ginecol* 1965; **11**(2): 131–47.

38. Borruto F, Chasen ST, Chervenak FA, Fedele L. The Vecchietti procedure for surgical treatment of vaginal agenesis: comparison of laparoscopy and laparotomy. *Int J Gynaecol Obstet* 1999; **64**(2): 153–58.

39. Christopoulos P, Cutner A, Vashisht A, Creighton SM. Laparoscopic sacrocolpopexy to treat prolapse of the neovagina created by vaginal dilation in Rokitansky syndrome. *J Pediatr Adolesc Gynecol* 2011; **24**(2): e33–34.

40. Davydov SN, Zhvitiashvili OD. Formation of vagina (colpopoiesis) from peritoneum of Douglas pouch. *Acta Chir Plast* 1974; **16**(1): 35–41.

41. Leblanc E, Bresson L, Merlot B, Puga M, Kridelka F, Tsunoda A, Narducci F. A simple laparoscopic procedure to restore a normal vaginal length after colpohysterectomy with large upper colpectomy for cervical and/or vaginal neoplasia. *J Minim Invasive Gynecol* 2016; **23**(1): 120–25.

42. Bouman MB, van Zeijl MC, Buncamper ME, Meijerink WJ, van Bodegraven AA, Mullender MG. Intestinal vaginoplasty revisited: a review of surgical techniques, complications, and sexual function. *J Sex Med* 2014; **11**(7): 1835–47.

43. Creatsas G, Deligeoroglou E, Christopoulos P. Creation of a neovagina after Creatsas modification of Williams vaginoplasty for the treatment of 200 patients with Mayer-Rokitansky-Kuster-Hauser syndrome. *Fertil Steril.* 2010; **94**(5): 1848–52.

44. Hung MJ, Wen MC, Hung CN, Ho ES, Chen GD, Yang VC. Tissue-engineered fascia from vaginal fibroblasts for patients needing reconstructive pelvic surgery. *Int Urogynecol J.* 2010; **21**(9): 1085–93.

45. Lloyd J, Crouch NS, Minto CL, Liao LM, Creighton SM. Female genital appearance: "normality" unfolds. *BJOG* 2005; **112**(5): 643–46.

46. Morcel K, Lavoué V, Jaffre F, Paniel BJ, Rouzier R. Sexual and functional results after creation of a neovagina in women with Mayer-Rokitansky-Kuster-Hauser syndrome: a comparison of nonsurgical and surgical procedures. *Eur J Obstet Gynecol Reprod Biol* 2013; **169**(2): 317–20.

47. Bean EJ, Mazur T, Robinson AD. Mayer-Rokitansky-Kuster-Hauser syndrome: sexuality, psychological effects, and quality of life. *J Pediatr Adolesc Gynecol* 2009; **22**(6): 339–46.

48. Friedler S, Grin L, Liberti G, Saar-Ryss B, Rabinson Y, Meltzer S. The reproductive potential of patients with Mayer-Rokitansky-Kuster-Hauser syndrome using gestational surrogacy: a systematic review. *Reprod Biomed Online* 2016; **32**(1): 54–61.

49. Raziel A, Friedler S, Gidoni Y, Ben Ami I, Strassburger D, Ron-El R. Surrogate in vitro fertilization outcome in typical and atypical forms of Mayer-Rokitansky-Kuster-Hauser syndrome. *Hum Reprod* 2012; **27**(1): 126–30.

50. Brännström M, Johannesson L, Bokström H, Kvarnström N, Mölne J, Dahm-Kähler P et al. Livebirth after uterus transplantation. *Lancet* 2015; **385**(9968): 607–16.

51. Brännström M. Uterus transplantation. *Curr Opin Organ Transplant* 2015; **20**(6): 621–28.

52. Farrell RM, Falcone T. Uterine transplant: new medical and ethical considerations. *Lancet* 2015; **385**(9968): 581–82.

Primary Amenorrhea in Pediatric and Adolescent Gynecology Practice
Disorders of Sex Development

Naomi S. Crouch and Gerard S. Conway

Background

Disorders of sex development (DSD) is an umbrella term encompassing those diagnoses where there is some discordance between expected and observed findings in terms of genetic sex, gonadal development, or appearance of the genitalia. This could include a female with 46XY karyotype, a female with testes, or a baby born with atypical genitalia representing either an over-virilized female or an under-virilized male. Such conditions were previously referred to as intersex, but terminology has changed following a consensus meeting between clinicians and patient groups [1]. Historical terms such as "pseudohermaphrodite" are technically inaccurate, widely disliked by patients and families and should not be used. Conditions are now referred to by their clinical descriptions. While the terminology has not been universally popular, there is no doubt that it has been widely accepted by the medical community and many patient groups [2].

Historically, the diagnosis of DSD was often cloaked in secrecy and shame, with the medical profession colluding in this [3]. Patients were not informed of their underlying diagnosis and alternative explanations were often offered, such as "diseased ovaries." While such strategies were often offered with good intentions, this practice is no longer acceptable, and clear openness with parents and ultimately individuals with DSD is a mandatory part of offering care. The model of caregiving has also changed with time, with the recognition that services need to be provided by a multidisciplinary team in a center of clinical expertise [4].

Embryology

To understand the spectrum of complex conditions that comprise DSDs, some knowledge of embryological development is required. The reproductive tract in the developing embryo consists of three main areas: the gonad, the internal genital tract, and the external genital and urinary opening.

The Gonad

Genetic sex in humans is determined at the point of conception to be either XX or XY. This leads to the formation of the gonadal ridge with an undifferentiated gonad that has the capacity to develop into either an ovary or a testis. Primordial germ cells migrate to the ridge and initiate sex differentiation. Sertoli cells (XY) or granulosa cells (XX) lead to the production of the sex steroids that is itself triggered by the presence (or not) of the sex-determining region of the Y chromosome – the SRY gene. The SRY initiates a series of genetic switches that promote cell differentiation. It is a highly complex process that ultimately leads to the expression of anti-Mullerian hormone (AMH), which regulates the development of the internal genital tract.

The Internal Genital Tract

The genital duct system consists of the Mullerian duct (MD) and the Woolfian duct (WD) systems that are a set of paired tubes that meet in the midline and continue caudally to the genital opening. The usual developmental pathway would be for the persistence of the MD resulting in usual female reproductive tract. However, the SRY leads to AMH expression that promotes regression of the MD and allows the WD to develop. The developing testis expresses androgens that act upon the androgen receptor (AR), which results in virilization of the genital tubercle into a penis enclosing the urethra, and the genital folds into the scrotum. In the absence of AMH, the MD develops into the Fallopian tubes, uterus and cervix, and upper two-thirds of the vagina. The MD meets the genital sinus at the site of the future hymen and allows the lower third of the vagina to become separate from the urethra with both opening onto the perineum.

If the gonads are dysgenetic, they cannot respond to the SRY gene and therefore will not express AMH. This allows the development of the MD, regression of the WD and results in the female phenotype.

The External Genital and Urinary Opening

The external genitalia develop from the cloacal membrane and form the genital tubercle, which develops into the clitoris and the cloacal fold forming the paired genital swellings that in turn form the labioscrotal folds. The cloacal fold forms the genital and anal folds resulting in separation between the anus and the urogenital sinus, which further divides into the urethra and the vagina. This sequence of events results in the usual three separate openings onto the female genital area.

Male external genital development is mediated by androgens, with virilization to females occurring in the presence of higher than usual androgens expressed. Conversely under-virilization may occur if androgens are not expressed or recognized by the developing male fetus. Interestingly, there appears to be a continuum in anatomical development between androgens and clitoral-to-urethra distance, with those with the lowest recognition of androgens showing the longest distance between structures [5].

Clinical Presentation

DSDs may be recognized at birth when a baby is born with atypical external genitalia. In some cases, a baby with marked virilization may be assigned male, only to return extremely unwell within a few days with an unrecognized diagnosis of salt-wasting congenital adrenal hyperplasia (CAH). DSDs may also present in childhood with the development of an inguinal hernia where the gonad has traveled into the labioscrotal fold. For many others, a DSD becomes apparent at puberty. This may be with the absence of periods, for those with an internal WD, or may be virilization to some degree for those with normal androgen receptor function [6].

Congenital Adrenal Hyperplasia

Congenital adrenal hyperplasia is the most common DSD with an incidence of 1:14000 births. It is an autosomal recessive condition, with several different subtypes; 90 percent of which are due to a deficiency of the enzyme 21-hydroxylase. The role of this enzyme is to enable cortisol and aldosterone production, as part of the delta 4 pathway, and its deficiency results in two effects: first, the development of a salt-wasting condition (Classical CAH), which is life threatening and results in death if not promptly recognized and treated with steroid replacement. Second, the precursors from the cortisol pathway lead to an excess of androgens causing external virilization of the female fetus.

As a result of androgenization in utero, the clitoris develops larger than usual and appears more prominent. The vagina is tucked inside the pelvis, "taking off" from the back of the urethra, leaving a single urogenital sinus opening on the perineum. The labial majora appear more rugose, having an appearance more typical of scrotal tissue.

Surgical Management

The advent of steroid treatment for those with salt-wasting CAH changed an immediately life-threatening condition into one with long-term management issues. Surgery to alter the genital area to a more typical female appearance therefore became a standard part of treatment. In more recent years, patients, families, and support groups have challenged this approach.

Indications for surgery include to allow penetrative intercourse, provide a conduit for menstruation, avoidance of urinary tract infections, and to reduce or avoid surgery in adolescence. In addition, it is often argued that a more typical female appearance to the genital area will promote parental bonding and reduce psychological distress for the child.

Surgical Approach

The mainstay of the surgical approach is to reduce the size of the clitoris and bring the vagina to open separately on the perineum to create a more typical female appearance. The clitoris consists of paired corpora with erectile tissue, with the neurovascular bundle running along the dorsal aspect. Nerves fan out around the glans, innervating the covering clitoral hood skin. The tail of the clitoris runs along the inner aspect of the pelvis on each side; therefore, the perineal clitoral tissue can reasonably be considered as the tip of the iceberg. The clitoris is highly innervated and forms a major component of female sexual pleasure and sensation. It has no other known function.

Surgical techniques have varied over the years, but the principle is to reduce the size and/or appearance of the clitoral tissue without long-term damage to function. Originally this involved removing the clitoral glans and clitoral hood, with the vagina being brought down to form a second perineal opening. An increasing appreciation of the importance of the clitoris in sexual pleasure and the role of female sexual function led to this approach being refined. The clitoral recession technique was developed to avoid removing any tissue, with the corporal bodies folded and sutured in place. This had the effect of reducing the prominence of the clitoral glans without dividing tissue. However, pain was a common complaint, particularly at the time of arousal, due to erectile tissue becoming trapped.

Further techniques involved dividing the clitoral hood skin, removing the corporal bodies, and setting the clitoral glans back into position. This was often combined with a vaginal procedure to draw the vaginal opening down to the perineum, with the clitoral skin being utilized to form labia minora. This is known as the one-stage procedure. Variations of this approach remain the mainstay of current surgery for those born with atypical genitalia.

Timing of Surgery

Current practice is for surgery to be performed in infancy, with proponents arguing the surgery is likely to be technically more straightforward due to the shorter distance involved. There may also be the effect of maternal estrogen, which promotes healing, and lasts for a few months after birth.

Results of Surgery

A few long-term outcome studies follow those who underwent childhood surgery. Cosmesis is reported variably, with surgeons often claiming excellent results. However, studies including assessments by researchers not part of the operating team have shown disappointing results [7]. There is no evidence that early childhood surgery protects against urinary tract infections [8]. In addition, studies have shown there is risk to sexual function with clitoral surgery [9]. The majority of individuals will still require surgical intervention at adolescence, which may not have been expected by those who have undergone one-stage surgery. There is also no evidence that childhood surgery promotes parental bonding or improves psychological outcomes for the child. In contrast,

some parents have written powerfully to suggest that of all the parenting concerns in having a child with congenital adrenal hyperplasia, the appearance of the genital area was not a major one [10].

Some form of surgery is likely to be needed to allow penetrative intercourse and facilitate tampon use. Obstruction to menstruation is unlikely in those who have not undergone surgery, and menstrual flow can occur through the common channel. Assessment may be made in early adolescence to ensure that no obstruction is present. Therefore, many clinicians would argue that surgery should be deferred until adolescence and would point to the importance of an individual being involved in the consent process [11]. A baby clearly cannot consent to cosmetic surgery, and the parents are being asked to make decisions on her behalf.

Surgery in adolescence will allow the endogenous effect of estrogen on the healing tissues, which is thought to be of importance in childhood surgery. There is no significant cohort of children who have not undergone childhood surgery, with the difficulty or otherwise of primary surgery in adolescence remaining largely unknown.

Controversies of Surgery

The surgical community appears to be in two camps; those who work within pediatric surgical surgery who think that early surgery in infancy is advisable, and those who work in adult surgical services who are often faced with the complications of childhood surgery. While the controversies of surgery for those with atypical genitalia are likely to continue to be hotly debated, some issues are incontrovertible.

- Surgery to the clitoral area is a cosmetic procedure
- Any surgery will interrupt nerve fibers
- Surgery will cause a risk to sexual function
- The child does not need a vagina
- The vagina may need surgery to allow menstrual flow and penetrative intercourse
- A larger than average clitoris is not a medical emergency

Complete Androgen Insensitivity Syndrome

Complete androgen insensitivity syndrome (CAIS) is the most common DSD for those with 46XY. It occurs in 1:40000 births and is an X-linked recessive condition. The androgen receptor (AR) gene is located at

Xq11–12. *AR* mutations result in variable resistance to signal transduction through the receptor that cannot respond to testosterone and its derivatives, meaning the external genitalia are unable to virilize. This results in a typical female appearance to the external genitalia with normal labia, clitoris, and urethra and lower third of the vagina. However, the gonads are fully functional testes that therefore express anti-Mullerian hormone, leading to the development of the Woolfian duct and regression of the Mullerian duct, as described earlier. The absence of the uterus and upper vagina therefore means the vagina is shortened and blind ending.

Diagnosis of CAIS

Those with CAIS typically present with primary amenorrhea with otherwise apparently normal secondary sexual characteristics. CAIS may also present in childhood with an inguinal hernia, with further investigations revealing this to be a testis. Breast development is normal, and girls are often tall, achieving male-typical height derived from the Y chromosome. However, there is usually no pubic or axillary hair development as this is mediated by the androgen receptor. In contrast to previous decades, current adolescents often desire hair removal and are less likely to be distressed by this feature.

Due to the genetic nature of the condition, on further enquiry it is not unusual to identify family members who may also have CAIS. However, 30 percent of cases result from do novo mutations and will have no family history. Because of the historical secrecy and stigma attached to all DSDs, information may be elusive, but the knowledge of an aunt or sister who was unable to have children may be significant.

A karyotype will be 46XY, and further blood tests will show normal functioning of all parts of the testosterone biosynthetic pathway. Targeted genetic studies will confirm a suspected mutation on the androgen receptor. Approximately 95 percent of clinical CAIS will have an identifiable androgen receptor mutation.

Gonadectomy

Gonadal malignancy risk for women with CAIS has traditionally been estimated to be around 5 percent, and the gonads are usually retained until later adolescence to allow completion of normal pubertal development, including breast development. Current practice would be to perform a laparoscopic gonadectomy in the late teenage years. Once the gonads are removed, girls need to take hormone replacement therapy (HRT) until the age of the natural menopause at 50. Recent work has suggested that the cancer risk in adults may be underestimated but accurate data are simply not available [12]. Historical studies may contain diagnostic inaccuracies, and participation in research studies may be flawed following an era of nondisclosure. Increasingly, some women may prefer to retain their gonads in preference to taking HRT long term, or to avoid the risk and inconvenience of surgery. These concerns need to be balanced against the unknown risks of deferring surgery and the difficulties in safe ongoing gonadal surveillance. This needs a clear discussion in adolescence and requires knowledge and understanding of the condition.

Management of Vaginal Hypoplasia

For those conditions where the Mullerian duct has not developed, such as CAIS, there will be vaginal hypoplasia, with a shortened blind-ending vagina and absence of the cervix and uterus. Various surgical procedures have been described, including skin grafts and bowel replacement. These are extensive and risk long-term complications including dryness, stenosis, and cancer development.

The accepted gold standard for development of the vagina is dilation therapy. This consists of using dilators that are pressed against the vaginal area for approximately 30 minutes per day. The area will gradually develop and dilators of increasing size may be used, with success rates of up to 85 percent achieved in developing a vagina suitable for intercourse. Once a length suitable for intercourse is achieved, provided this is taking place at least weekly, no further treatment is indicated. For episodes of coital infrequency, use of the dilator weekly will maintain vaginal length.

Studies have shown it takes up to 6 months of dilator therapy for the developing vagina to be comfortable for penetrative intercourse, and success is strongly related to compliance [13]. Vaginal dilation has also been shown to be the most cost-effective strategy, as well as enabling the woman to choose the timing of treatment, and to have control over progression [14]. However, while it may seem clinically simplistic and effective, many psychological barriers may prevent success. Involvement of a psychologist in treatment is essential to guide a woman as to the timing of starting treatment, and also to provide psychological support through the process.

When dilators are not successful, a Vecchietti procedure may be offered. This is a laparoscopic procedure whereby a small plastic bead is placed in the vaginal canal, and threads are passed up through the abdominal cavity and out onto the abdomen. These are then attached to a mechanism that can lift the vagina by drawing on the bead. Approximately 1-cm length may be achieved each day, resulting in a potentially functioning vagina over a week or so. Dilators would need to be used on a weekly basis after the procedure to maintain vaginal length, unless the individual were sexually active with a partner. This would now represent the main surgical alternative, but as with dilators, psychological management is crucial to support a successful outcome.

46XY DSD

Testosterone Biosynthetic Defect Diagnoses

As described earlier, sex determination is a complex process requiring intact genetic pathways, but also biochemical pathways. Several rarer DSD conditions are caused by enzyme deficiencies in the pathway of testosterone synthesis. Individuals have an XY karyotype, and as there is an intact androgen receptor some degree of virilization will occur. The Woolfian duct will have developed with regression of the Mullerian duct. Depending on the degree of virilization, a baby may present with atypical genitalia and be considered as an under-virilized male, or virilized female child.

Once a testosterone biosynthetic defect diagnosis is suspected, biochemical tests assessing the ratios between each hormone will usually indicate the likely diagnosis. For example, 5alpha reductase is the enzyme catalyzing the reaction between testosterone and the much more active dihydrotestosterone (DHT) resulting in a 10:1 ratio. If the testosterone: DHT ratio is less than this, a diagnosis of 5alpha reductase deficiency is likely. Another enzyme defect impairs the conversion of androstenedione to testosterone. Mutations of the *HSD17B3* gene result in deficiency of 17-beta hydroxysteroid dehydrogenase with the biochemical marker of serum testosterone: androstenedione ratio <0.8 [15,16].

Genetic studies can identify causal mutations in the majority of individuals with 46XY DSD. Accuracy in diagnosis is of great importance to individuals and clinicians alike. It is difficult to guide parents and patients without a clear idea of likely outcomes. It also does not allow individuals to take part in research studies, access peer support, or give the wider family information about a potential genetic carrier status for apparently unaffected individuals.

If the diagnosis is not made at birth or in childhood, individuals may present with further virilization at puberty with enlargement of the clitoris, deepening of the voice, and male-pattern hair growth, in which case the diagnostic steps presented earlier are followed.

Dysgenetic Gonads

Some DSD conditions result from dysgenetic and hence nonfunctioning gonads, leading to a failure to enter puberty. Individuals will present with primary amenorrhea and delayed secondary sexual characteristics. A significant difference with those with dysgenetic gonads, such as those with 46XY complete gonadal dysgenesis, is that AMH will not have been expressed in utero. This results in the Mullerian duct persisting, and individuals would have a uterus, cervix, and upper and lower vagina.

Girls with gonadal dysgenesis will need to undergo pubertal induction to allow normal development and will need long-term hormone replacement therapy. The modern approach would be to use estrogen patches that allow continuous slow release of estrogen [17]. Progestogen is added once periods establish. Puberty induction is a highly specialized intervention and should be offered by a specialist endocrinologist.

Surgical Management

Role of Gonadectomy

Once a diagnosis of a 46XY DSD has been made, it is likely that a gonadectomy is indicated. For those conditions where the gonads are dysgenetic in the presence of a Y chromosome, such as Swyer syndrome or 45X/46XY mixed gonadal dysgenesis (Turner Mosaic), the risk of malignancy is in the order of 30 percent [18]. For this reason, current management recommends gonadectomy at the time of diagnosis, which often occurs in adolescents presenting with delayed puberty. In addition, gonadectomy may also be required reasonably urgently to prevent further virilization in adolescent girls with conditions such as 5-alpha reductase deficiency or 17-beta hydroxysteroid dehydrogenase deficiency where there is androgen receptor function. Continued testosterone production will therefore result in further virilization that may not be reversible.

Vaginal Development

For those with 46XY complete gonadal dysgenesis, the Mullerian duct will have developed completely. Once puberty has been achieved, no further treatment would be needed to allow menstrual flow and subsequently penetrative vaginal intercourse.

Where there is a diagnosis of a 46XY testosterone biosynthetic pathway dysfunction, a short vaginal passage usually exists. This is of varying length, and dilator therapy may be offered. As no uterus is present, there is no urgency with this, and it may be offered when the girl chooses. As with those with CAIS, psychological support is mandatory for this process.

Fertility

Options for fertility vary according to the presence or absence of the uterus. For instance, women with 46XY gonadal dysgenesis usually have intact uterine function and can achieve normal pregnancy using oocyte donation. In this way, pregnancy options are the same as for all women with ovarian insufficiency.

For women with an absent or vestigial uterus, the only fertility option is with surrogacy and the opportunity to use one's own gametes will vary according to the genetic subtype. For instance, for individuals with 5-alpha reductase deficiency, there is a possibility of retrieving viable sperm from the testes at the time of gonadectomy with a view to long-term sperm cryopreservation. Theoretically, some cryopreserved sperm could be used with a donor oocyte and subsequent surrogacy. These issues are increasingly of consideration for women approaching gonadectomy. It is likely, however, that successful sperm retrieval is limited to individuals at the male end of the clinical spectrum because a significant degree of enzyme function is required to generate intra-testicular testosterone to allow for maturation of sperm. An illustration of this comes from complete androgen insensitivity where it is only primitive spermatids that are generally found on histological examination of testes, and there is no record of viable sperm being retrieved [19].

Long-term Health Outcomes

Little data record the natural history of most DSDs in later adult life. Specific conditions have associated syndromic features that require attention. For instance, NR5A1 mutations may have concurrent adrenal insufficiency that may be subclinical and have to be tested for specifically.

Long-term monitoring for women with the DSD is best undertaken in a multidisciplinary service specializing in this range of conditions. The main reason for this is to address the common frustration experienced by women with DSD when confronting doctors who know little about the condition and have no experience in gender issues, sexual function, or estrogen replacement issues. Monitoring of estrogen replacement should proceed along conventional lines as recommended for women with ovarian insufficiency.

Endocrine Management

Estrogen deficiency between ages 12 and 50 should be addressed as soon as it is identified. For females identified at a young age, induction of puberty using transdermal patches containing estradiol should proceed along established guidelines as discussed in Chapter 8B. The preferred agent for long-term estrogen replacement is estradiol, which can be administered by oral and transdermal routes. Usual dose range for estradiol is 2–4 mg daily and for the transdermal patch 50–100 μg daily. The individualized dose of estrogen is determined mainly by symptoms and overall well-being, taking into account bone density measurements that should be undertaken approximately every 5 years.

Other forms of estrogen such as ethinylestradiol and conjugated equine estrogens are not recommended because of their higher risk of thrombosis compared to estradiol. Transdermal route of administration is preferred because of the lower risk of thrombosis compared to oral estradiol, although very young women prefer oral estradiol because it is more discreet [20,21].

Women with an intact uterus such as those with 46XY gonadal dysgenesis (Swyer syndrome) require progestogen, which can be administered on a sequential basis for 12 days of each month or as a low-dose continuous progestogen without withdrawal bleeds. An intrauterine levonorgestral-releasing device is an alternative method of providing endometrial protection with progestogen.

Women with complete androgen insensitivity syndrome with retained gonads do not usually require sex steroid support because endogenous testosterone provides sufficient estrogen through aromatization to allow for more bone density and well-being. Women with CAIS have an additional option to use testosterone supplements either in the form of topical gel application or a depot injection. Some women with CAIS believe that testosterone is a benefit because it returns the endocrine milieu to what existed prior to gonadectomy and also because they consider testosterone to be benefit for well-being. No long-term data are available regarding the use of testosterone in this manner; neither is there any theoretical reason why testosterone supplements should not be offered to women with CAIS.

Sex steroid replacement is usually continued until about age 50, although some women may choose to continue beyond that age if symptoms of estrogen deficiency are sufficiently disabling. Extrapolating from women using estrogen replacement after menopause, there may be an increased risk of breast cancer with exposure to estrogen over age 55, and that small risk has to be balanced against symptomatic benefit.

Psychology

The scientific understanding of DSDs has changed immeasurably over the past two decades, but with this comes the continued and increasing need for psychological support for families and girls diagnosed with a DSD. Once considered as an afterthought, the role of psychology is slowly being seen as essential and underpins the whole of care for those with a DSD [4,22].

A diagnosis is often made in childhood or adolescence with a planned transition of care to adult services required. However, the all-encompassing clinical care from pediatric services is often not matched in adult services with many of those with DSDs struggling to access the lifelong multidisciplinary care that is needed.

Recent work assessed the urgency of the clinical needs of those adolescents with a DSD who were transitioning to adult services [22]. While no urgent issues were identified regarding medical or surgical care, psychological issues were consistently seen as the most important and pressing need of individuals, yet they are often the area of care that is least likely to be funded.

Issues that adolescents are confronting include vaginal treatment, gonadectomy, hormone replacement therapy, and future fertility options. Adolescents will be involved in the decisions for their care, which may at times seem counterintuitive to parents and clinicians. For those who had a diagnosis made in childhood, a further challenge is the disclosing of medical knowledge to the individual. This is performed in a graded way and may take many months or years. Parents have often been worried or even fearful about this process and will also need care and compassion in the process.

The emergence of peer support groups has been further encouraged with the growth of social media. Many groups offer support to families and individuals in a manner that is different but complementary to that offered by clinicians.

Further information is available in Chapter 12.

Conclusions

From a past of secrecy and shame, the modern management of DSDs is now patient and family centered. Individuals require lifelong care, and an improvement in accuracy of diagnosis and openness with clinicians has facilitated information for patients and the development of many research studies. The role of a multidisciplinary team in pediatrics should be matched by that in adult services and must include a psychologist as a core member of the group.

References

1. Hughes IA, Houk C. Ahmed SF, Lee PA. Lawson Wilkins Pediatric Endocrine Society (LWPES)/ European Society for Pediatric Endocrinology (ESPE) Consensus Group. Consensus statement on the management of intersex disorders. *J Ped Urol* 2006; **2**(3): 148–62.

2. Pasterski V, Prentice P, Hughes IA. Impact of the consensus statement and the new DSD classification system *Best Practice & Research Clinical Endocrinology & Metabolism*, 2010; **24**(2): 187–95.

3. Once a dark secret. Anon. *BMJ* 1994; **308**: 542.

4. Horm Res Pediatr. 2016; **85**(3): 158–80. doi: 10.1159/ 000442975. Epub 2016 Jan 28. Global Disorders of Sex Development Update since 2006: Perceptions, Approach and Care. Lee PA, Nordenström A, Houk CP, Ahmed SF, Auchus R, Baratz A et al.; Global DSD Update Consortium.

5. Crouch N, Michala L, Creighton S, Conway G. Androgen-dependent measurements of female genitalia

in women with complete androgen insensitivity syndrome. *BJOG* 2011; **118**: 84–87.

6. Berra M, Liao LM, Creighton SM, Conway GS. Long-term health issues of women with XY karyotype. *Maturitas* 2010; **65**(2): 172–78. doi: 10.1016/j.maturitas.2009.12.004. Epub 2010 Jan 15. Review. PubMed PMID: 20079588.

7. Michala L, Liao LM, Wood D, Conway GS, Creighton SM. Practice changes in childhood surgery for ambiguous genitalia? *J Pediatr Urol* 2014; **10**(5): 934–39.

8. Nabhan ZM, Rick RC, Eugster EA. Urinary tract infections in children with congenital adrenal hyperplasia. *J Pediatr Surg* 2004; **39**: 1030–33.

9. Crouch NS, Liao LM, Woodhouse CRJ, Conway GS, Creighton SM. Sexual function and genital sensitivity following feminizing genitoplasty for congenital adrenal hyperplasia. *J Urol* 2008; **179**: 634–38.

10. Magritte E. Working together in placing the long term interests of the child at the heart of the DSD evaluation. *J Pediatr Urol* 2012; **8**(6): 571–75.

11. Liao LM, Wood D, Crieghton SM. Parental choice on normalising cosmetic genital surgery. *BMJ* 2015; **351**: h5124.

12. Deans R, Creighton SM, Liao LM, Conway GS. Timing of gonadectomy in adult women with complete androgen insensitivity syndrome (CAIS): patient preferences and clinical evidence. *Clin Endocrinol (Oxf)* 2012; **76**(6): 894–98.

13. Ismail-Pratt IS, Bikoo M, Liao LM, Conway GS, Creighton SM. Normalization of the vagina by dilator treatment alone in Complete Androgen Insensitivity Syndrome and Mayer-Rokitansky-Kuster-Hauser Syndrome. *Hum Reprod* 2007; **22**(7): 2020–24.

14. Routh JC, Laufer MR, Cannon GM, Jr., Diamond DA, Gargollo PC. Management strategies for Mayer-Rokitansky-Kuster-Hauser related vaginal agenesis: a cost-effectiveness analysis. *J Urol* 2010; **184**(5): 2116–21.

15. Berra M, Williams EL, Muroni B, Creighton SM, Honour JW, Rumsby G, Conway GS. Recognition of 5α-reductase-2 deficiency in an adult female 46XY DSD clinic. *Eur J Endocrinol.* 2011; **164**(6): 1019–25. doi: 10.1530/EJE-10-0930. Epub 2011 Mar 15. PubMed PMID: 21402750.

16. Phelan N, Williams EL, Cardamone S, Lee M, Creighton SM, Rumsby G, Conway GS. Screening for mutations in 17β-hydroxysteroid dehydrogenase and androgen receptor in women presenting with partially virilised 46,XY disorders of sex development. *Eur J Endocrinol.* 2015; **172**(6): 745–51. doi: 10.1530/EJE-14-0994. Epub 2015 Mar 4. PubMed PMID: 25740850.

17. Conway GS. Sex steroid treatment for pubertal induction and replacement in the adolescent girl (scientific impact paper no. 40). Royal College of Obstetricians and Gynaecologists 2013.

18. Pleskacova J, Hersmus R, Oosterhuis JW, Setyawati BA, Faradz SM, Cools M, et al. Tumor risk in disorders of sex development. *Sex Dev* 2010; **4**(4–5): 259–69.

19. Kang HJ, Imperato-McGinley J, Zhu YS, Rosenwaks Z. The effect of 5α-reductase-2 deficiency on human fertility. *Fertil Steril.* 2014; **101**(2): 310–16.

20. Smith NL, Blondon M, Wiggins KL, Harrington LB, van Hylckama Vlieg A, Floyd JS et al. Lower risk of cardiovascular events in postmenopausal women taking oral estradiol compared with oral conjugated equine estrogens. *JAMA Intern Med.* 2014; **174**(1): 25–31.

21. Weill A, Dalichampt M, Raguideau F, Ricordeau P, Blotière PO, Rudant J et al. Low dose oestrogen combined oral contraception and risk of pulmonary embolism, stroke, and myocardial infarction in five million French women: cohort study. *BMJ.* 2016; **10**:353: i2002.

22. Crouch NS, Creighton SM. Transition of care for adolescents with disorders of sex development. *Nat Rev Endocrinol.* 2014; **10**(7): 436–42.

23. Liao LM, Tacconelli E, Wood D, Conway G, Creighton SM. Adolescent girls with disorders of sex development: A needs analysis of transitional care. *J Pediatr Urol* 2010; **6**(6): 609–13.

Urinary Problems in Pediatric and Adolescent Gynecology Practice
Incontinence and Lower Urinary Tract Symptoms

Alun Williams and Anette Jacobsen

Introduction

Genitourinary problems in childhood are common and present variably across the spectrum of primary and secondary care services. In particular, urinary tract infection (UTI) and wetting are common in both boys and girls, more so in girls.

Congenital abnormalities that predispose to infection and incontinence are described in more detail in Chapter 9B and elsewhere in this book. Anomalies such as spinal dysraphism, duplication of the upper urinary tract with associated ureteric ectopia or reflux, and urethral and urogenital sinus abnormalities can be subtle and easy to miss without formal anatomical assessment. Most congenital abnormalities, however, present in utero or early in childhood.

Urinary Tract Infection

Up to 10 percent of girls (and 3 percent of boys) will have had a UTI during childhood [1]. The incidence of infection falls with increasing age during childhood. Interestingly, UTIs in infant girls are less common than in boys, reflecting the marked increased association in this age group with congenital uropathies, vesicoureteric reflux (VUR) being the most common. Beyond infancy, UTI becomes much more common in girls. About one in four infants treated for UTI has a recurrent infection. In older girls the risk of recurrence becomes much higher: about 60 percent will experience a recurrent UTI.

Escherichia coli is by far the most common causative organism. Other organisms, such as *Proteus, Enterococcus, Klebsiella*, and *Pseudomonas* occur. Fungi and viruses rarely cause problems in immunecompetent children. Predisposing "host" factors include congenital upper tract problems such as vesicoureteric reflux or renal and ureteric dilatation, incomplete bladder emptying, and dysfunctional voiding. A careful history will include details of antenatal concerns, postnatal voiding history (including toilet training, frequency of voiding, character of voiding such as interrupted stream and abdominal straining, for example). Detailed history of bowel function follows with examination for palpable masses including fecal loading. Careful examination of the perineum and examination of the spine and lower limbs for signs of occult spinal dysraphism, such as a hairy, fatty, or hemangiomatous patch on the back or sacral spine, complete assessment.

The symptoms of UTI are often rather vague. In infants and preverbal children, vomiting is the most common presenting feature. Fever is often present and in the context of an unwell baby, urine culture is mandatory. More classical features such as frequency, urgency, meatal or abdominal pain, and wetting tend to be more common in older children. There is very often a history of infrequent passage of hard stool, irregular bowel habit, or soiling from overflow incontinence. These complaints may have been masquerading under the umbrella term of "constipation" as part of a history for UTI. A discharge, which may or may not be vaginal in origin, and perineal soreness may be other common associated symptoms.

A urine specimen needs to be collected carefully. Most children who can void "on demand" are able to give a reliable midstream urine sample. In babies, urine is best collected by a clean catch – although this is sometimes frustrating. Collection bags are commonly used but especially in baby girls are prone to result in contaminated specimens. Samples need to be delivered fresh (although refrigeration overnight in a sterile container is probably acceptable). In unwell children, catheter specimens or suprapubic aspirates in babies are the best and most reliable means of collection.

The gold standard of diagnosis of UTI is on the basis of formal culture of a pure growth of an organism with a colony count of $>10^5$ organisms/ml associated with white cells. Sensitivities are usually generated with organism culture.

The treatment of a UTI depends ultimately on the sensitivity. If possible it is good practice to base antibiotic prescription on laboratory culture. There is a significant (and highly geographically variable) pattern of resistance of common organisms to antibiotics such as trimethoprim, penicillins, or cephalosporins. However an empirical treatment with a broad spectrum antibiotic is sometimes needed.

Subsequent investigation and management depend on the clinical context of the UTI. Most uncomplicated *E. coli* UTIs in otherwise well children will not be associated with an underlying problem and can be safely treated as a "one-off." Recurrent UTI, unusual organisms, or infections in infancy demand a more considered approach; these are the children requiring imaging and assessment of their kidneys in more detail.

Guidelines are helpful for precise investigation and treatment. In the UK, the National Institute for Health and Care Excellence (NICE) has established evidence-based guidelines [2].

Some children go on to develop recurrent infection despite normal investigation of their urinary tracts. This group includes more girls than boys, and anatomical abnormalities are very rare. Assessment of stored and voided volumes (to assess residual urine volume) and uroflowmetry can sometimes identify dysfunctional voiding (see later). These children frequently have associated bowel disturbance that needs to be treated aggressively. Prophylactic antibiotics may be considered empirically but vigilance for resistance is important.

Incontinence

Uncontrolled leakage of urine per urethra may happen continuously or be intermittent. It is important to remember the clinical context, as well as the age of the child. Normal infants void in a manner akin to reflex – many times per day, and so for a baby or toddler in diapers this definition of incontinence is unhelpful. One symptom that can raise suspicion is a watery vaginal discharge in a child who has progressed to wearing underwear. Collection of urine on voiding into the vagina can occur occasionally even in girls with normal genital anatomy. This can also indicate a urogenital sinus abnormality and can sometimes indicate an ectopic ureter. The distinction between daytime symptoms and symptoms purely at night is also important.

Daytime wetting is very common [3]. Three percent of 7-year-old girls (2 percent of boys) have at least once-a-week symptoms of wetting. Of these between a third and a half will have nighttime symptoms too. Bedwetting without daytime symptoms (primary monosymptomatic nocturnal enuresis – or simply "enuresis" now, according to the International Children's Continence Society [4]) is also very common. Up to one in ten of 7-year-old children wet three or more nights per week.

Symptoms of wetting occur in such heterogeneous conditions that it is unhelpful to consider the broad group together. Classification of symptoms may be helpful in suggesting the presence of overactive bladder – namely that urgency and frequency raise suspicion. The issue of "stress" symptoms is less in children. Symptoms precipitated by coughing, sneezing, high-impact exercise, or laughing are still far more likely to be as a consequence of overactive bladder than of true stress incontinence. As indicated later, stress incontinence might be due to neuropathic muscle weakness in association with a spinal cord problem. Primary myopathies are exceedingly rare. One condition perhaps worthy of mention is the congenital short urethra. This can only be assessed reliably at cytsourethroscopy. It is probably a variant ("forme fruste") of epispadias.

The importance of clinical examination for UTI is mirrored for the group with wetting. Detailed abdominal examination might reveal masses or palpable kidneys or bladder, or palpable stool in the colon or rectum. Again it is important to examine the spine for features of an occult dysraphism. Small dimples and pits in the coccygeal region are common, and a dilemma may often arise as to whether an MRI (which may require general anesthesia in small children) is needed to exclude a tethered cord or spinal dysraphism. In the context of incontinence, it is difficult to dismiss any abnormality that is known to associate with an underlying spinal problem. The presence of flat buttocks, asymmetrical skin creases, or a palpable abnormality of the sacrum (such as its absence) may indicate sacral dysgenesis or agenesis. Abnormal lower limb power, reflexes, sensation, or abnormal perineal sensation needs further investigation with a view to spinal imaging.

Examination of the perineum is crucial. Labial fusion is easy to spot. A single anterior perineal orifice distinct from the anus might point toward the presence of a urogenital sinus abnormality. An abnormally sited

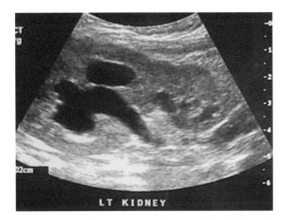

Figure 9A.1a Ultrasound image showing duplex kidney with dilated upper pole

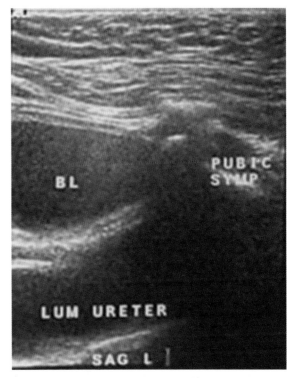

Figure 9A.1b Ultrasound image showing ectopic upper polar ureter passing behind the bladder

anus might suggest an anorectal malformation, such as a variant of a cloacal abnormality. In female epispadias (which is exceptionally rare with an incidence of 1:40000), two halves of the clitoral corporal bodies are widely spaced with a bladder neck opening in the perineum. These abnormalities, whilst rare, may however have gone previously undiagnosed if the child had never been examined. Cloacal abnormalities and conditions on the exstrophy/epispadias spectrum are considered in Chapter 9B.

Investigation of incontinence revolves around defining anatomy by means of physical examination followed by imaging, and defining the ability of the bladder to store and empty by recording volumes, flows, and pressures.

Ultrasound is a reliable, relatively noninvasive and inexpensive means of assessing the kidneys and bladder. It has more utility in children because of its ease of use. MRI and CT are valuable in certain circumstances, but ultrasound is the mainstay of pediatric urinary tract imaging.

Duplication anomalies of the kidney are quite reliably detected on ultrasound (Figure 9A.1a), as is pelvicalyceal dilatation. A duplex kidney, where there is complete duplication (two collecting systems, two ureters along their entire length) consistently has its upper pole drain more inferiorly and medially than its lower pole. This may be insignificant if both ureters drain into the bladder. However, if the upper pole moiety drains below the bladder outlet (Figure 9A.1b), it will cause incontinence. In a girl this will most commonly be drainage paraurethrally or into the vagina. The pattern of wetting is quite characteristic – namely, "continent incontinence" where there is a virtually constant dribble or drip of urine despite apparently normal voids. This is easily explained. The bladder fills and empties normally, but the ectopic ureter usually only subtends a kidney moiety that is poorly functioning and rather dysplastic. Renography might be needed to demonstrate renal function to guide management, but definitive treatment for an ectopic ureter with a dysplastic upper moiety of a duplex kidney is disconnection of the ureter (either by partial nephrectomy or more recently ureteric ligation [5]).

Bilateral duplex systems with bilateral upper pole ectopics are very rare. Bilateral ectopia in single systems is even rarer, but regrettably a much more formidable reconstructive challenge – these very abnormal urinary tracts usually require augmentation cystoplasty in addition to outlet procedures for incontinence.

Another association of duplex systems is an ureterocele. Again, ureterocoeles tend to be associated with the upper pole moiety; when they are intravesical, they tend to be more medial and inferior to the normal ureteric insertion. If large there is a risk of causing intermittent obstruction of the bladder neck –

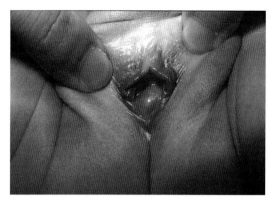

Figure 9A.1c Prolapsing ureterocele (ectopic ureterocele subtending upper pole ureter of duplex kidney)

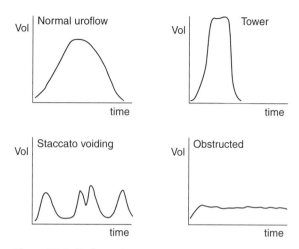

Figure 9A.2 Uroflowmetry curves

or even prolapse through the urethral meatus (Figure 9A.1c). This phenomenon is most common in neonates and requires decompression of the ureterocele (or later excision).

Bladder capacity can be assessed with ultrasound – and corroborated by recording voided volumes. Generally, the residual urine volume should be no more than 10 percent of capacity. Beyond infancy, the predicted bladder capacity can be estimated by this formula (among others):

$$\text{capacity (ml)} = (\text{age in years} + 2) \times 30 \text{ ml} \quad [6]$$

Urine flow rate (uroflowmetry) is a helpful noninvasive investigation. To yield a meaningful assessment, it does require the child to store urine that can be voided on demand. The configuration of the curve can aid definition of a voiding problem. Figure 9A.2 shows some examples of typical uroflow curves. Very rapid voiding over a short period of time (a "tower" configuration) can indicate overactive bladder. A "staccato" flow indicates dysfunctional voiding with dys-synergic contraction of the outlet. A flat and prolonged curve indicates obstruction – in itself quite rare in girls.

Urodynamics involves the transduction of bladder (P_{ves}) and intra-abdominal (P_{abd}) pressures to calculate the pressure generated by the detrusor muscle (P_{det}). This is done by filling the bladder via a urethral or suprapubic catheter at a predetermined rate, or in certain circumstances (so-called natural fill) to fill from the kidneys as normal. The abdominal pressure is measured using a rectal balloon catheter. Figure 9A.3a illustrates catheter placement. The true detrusor pressure is then calculated ($P_{ves} - P_{abd} = P_{Det}$).

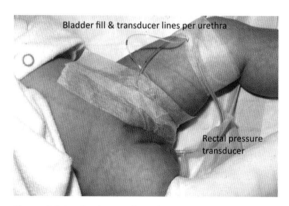

Figure 9A.3a Urodynamic line placement

Most useful is video urodynamics whereby the bladder is filled using radio-opaque contrast with concomitant radiological screening during the filling and voiding phase. The anatomy of the bladder, reflux into the ureters, descent of the bladder base, and the urethra can then be assessed in real time as the bladder fills and empties. EMG patch electrodes in the perineum can be placed to investigate the pelvic floor muscle activity. By definition, urodynamics are invasive and in children need to be considered carefully.

Overactive Bladder

Urgency (whether or not associated with wetting), frequency, and small voided volumes are the hallmarks of overactive bladder. In infants, bladders are, by definition, overactive, and so symptoms might sometimes be regarded as on a continuum of normal. Urodynamics

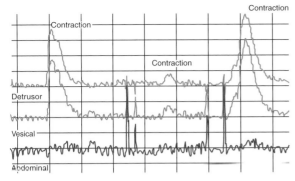

Figure 9A.3b Cystometrogram showing detrusor overactivity

might demonstrate true detrusor overactivity with contractions (Figure 9A.3b). The mainstay of treatment is with anticholinergics. Intradetrusor *Botulinum* toxin injection is gaining ground as a valuable (but short-lived – 6 months or so) treatment.

Dysfunctional Voiding

The typical uroflowmetry profile of dysfunctional voiding is shown in Figure 9A.2 (staccato). The child has repeated contractions of the outlet during voiding, which might be seen on the EMG recording during urodynamics. Residual urine (and predisposition to UTI) is common, as are more subtle consequences of intermittent obstruction – bladder wall thickening and impaired compliance of detrusor. There is a risk of compromise to the kidneys with this condition. Initial conservative regimens of treatment such as regular and timed voids and double voids to treat residual urine can be helpful. Biofeedback is a useful adjunct when it is available as this allows the child to become aware of pelvic floor contraction.

Underactive Bladder

The definition of underactive bladder used to be synonymous with "infrequent voiding" or "lazy bladder" but seems to be an entity whereby the bladder is able to store very large volumes and generate inefficient voiding. Treatment with regular and timed voids and sometimes intermittent catheterization might be helpful.

Giggle Incontinence

As mentioned earlier, wetting (or symptoms of urgency) on laughing usually associate more with overactive bladder, but a rare entity of pure giggle incontinence occurs with otherwise normal bladder function – and laughing can precipitate a full void. It remains very poorly understood, and long-standing evidence suggests that it is a centrally mediated phenomenon of arousal mechanisms. It seems to have a preponderance in families and is notoriously difficult to treat. CNS stimulants, such as methylphenidate, have been documented as being variably useful.

Vaginal Voiding (Vaginal Reflux)

Vaginal voiding is a phenomenon of prepubertal girls. There may be associated labial adhesions. The symptom pattern is often that of wetting within a few minutes of a void. Treatment revolves around emptying urine that has collected in the vagina – such as a post-void valsalva. Labial adhesions can be treated by topical corticosteroids or estrogens.

Nocturnal Enuresis

Nocturnal enuresis is a common condition in girls and boys (up to one in ten 7 year olds). It has a strong family history basis – but no clear single mechanism of inheritance [7]. There may be impaired bladder capacity. Rarely is there a true problem with urine concentrating ability, demonstrated by measuring urine osmolalities.

There are interesting associated risk factors, which predict poorer outcome from treatment rather than guide treatment. Ex-prematurity, reactive airways disease (asthma), attention-deficit hyperactivity disorder, and autistic spectrum disorder and sleep apnea are examples. The latter can be addressed sometimes by adenotonsillectomy [8].

Mainstays of treatment of enuresis are withholding fluid before bed, enuresis alarms, and vasopressin analogues. Sometimes combining treatments can be help. Adjunct anticholinergics can be helpful. The prevalence of enuresis falls over time with resolution. On average one child in twelve will be dry in 12 months. About 2 percent will persist with symptoms into adulthood and may be a group with more severe symptoms per se [9].

Neuropathic Conditions

Among this heterogeneous group, the most common condition is spina bifida – and other dysraphic conditions, although spinal injury, tumors, and pelvic surgery can predispose to neuropathic bladder and bowel.

The assessment and treatment are beyond the scope of this chapter, but clinical examination to rule out (or confirm) a possible neuropathic condition as described earlier is important. Treatment involves anticholinergics to mitigate overactive detrusor contractions and improve compliance, catheterization to aid voiding, and regular surveillance of the kidneys to preempt upper tract deterioration. Patients are best served by a multidisciplinary service as they often have coexisting spinal, orthopedic, and neurosurgical problems.

Bladder Pain

Again, a heterogeneous selection of conditions causes distress. The formerly used term "interstitial cystitis" has been superseded by the term "painful bladder syndrome." There are medical strategies for analgesia in the form of oral and intravesical preparations. Surgery is regarded as a last resort. One increasingly common condition with the ascent of the use of ketamine as a recreational drug is a debilitating condition with progressive fibrosis of the bladder [10].

Urinary Retention

Urinary retention is reported increasingly among teenagers and young adults. There are some conditions described eponymously (the exemplar is Fowler's syndrome based on characteristic neurophysiology findings in the periurethral muscles), although increasingly a spectrum of comorbidity is recognized [11]. This group of women can have challenging and refractory symptoms. Urinary drainage, usually by means of catheterization, is the mainstay of treatment. It is crucial to exclude structural causes (such as pelvic malignancy), neuropathic conditions, and central demyelinating disease.

References

1. Selekman RE, Allen IE, Copp HL. Determinants of practice patterns in pediatric UTI management. *J Pediatr Urol* 2016 Jul 5. **pii**: S1477–5131(16)30136-X. doi: 10.1016/j.jpurol.2016.05.036. [Epub ahead of print]

2. NICE Clinical Guideline Urinary tract infection: diagnosis, treatment and long-term management of urinary tract infection in children. 2007. Downloaded from http://guidance.nice.org.uk/CG54

3. Thomas DFM, Duffy PG, Rickwood, AMK., eds. *Essentials of Pediatric Urology*, 2nd ed. London: Informa Healthcare, 2008.

4. Austin PF, Bauer SB, Bower W et al. The standardization of terminology of lower urinary tract function in children and adolescents: update report from the standardization committee of the International Children's Continence Society. *Neurourol Urodyn* 2016; **35**(4): 471–81.

5. Romao RL, Figueroa V, Salle JL et al. Laparoscopic ureteral ligation (clipping): a novel, simple procedure for pediatric urinary incontinence due to ectopic ureters associated with non-functioning upper pole renal moieties. *J Pediatr Urol* 2014; **10**(6): 1089–94.

6. Koff SA. Estimating bladder capacity in children. *Urology* 1983; **21**: 248.

7. Loeys B, Hoebeke P, Raes A et al. Does monosymptomatic enuresis exist? A molecular genetic exploration of 32 families with enuresis/incontinence. *BJU Int* 2002; **90**: 76–83.

8. Basha S, Bialowas C, Ende K, Szeremeta W. Effectiveness of adenotonsillectomy in the resolution of nocturnal enuresis secondary to obstructive sleep apnea. *Laryngoscope* 2005; **115**: 1101–13.

9. Yeung CK, Sihoe JDY, Sit FKY et al. Characteristics of primary nocturnal enuresis in adults: an epidemiological study. *BJU Int* 2004; **93**: 341–45.

10. Chu PS, Ma WK, Wong SC et al. The destruction of the lower urinary tract by ketamine abuse: a new syndrome? *BJU Int* 2008; **102**(11): 1616–22.

11. Hoeritzauer I, Stone J, Fowler C et al. Fowler's syndrome of urinary retention: a retrospective study of co-morbidity. *Neurourol Urodyn* 2016; **35**(5): 601–3.

Urinary Problems in Pediatric and Adolescent Gynecology Practice
Congenital Anomalies and Bladder Diversion

Lesley Breech and Dan Wood

Introduction

Children and adolescents with congenital anomalies of the genitourinary tract have complex care needs and are often seen by a number of providers in the pediatric setting. The first priority will be preservation of life and then function. In this setting, ensuring a safe urinary tract to preserve renal function is a high priority; social continence (both fecal and urinary) is also high on the list. In the early years, it is nearly impossible to expect pediatric providers to account for all aspects of long-term function and late effects on fertility and sexual function. Reproductive outcomes remain poorly understood in many complex conditions. Historically, the pediatric urologist and surgeon have been the primary caregivers. While some have broad long-term experience, many do not. They often lack expertise relating to puberty, menarche, and reproduction, missing opportunities to intervene and avoid negative sequelae (such as pain, additional surgery, or reduced fertility). As overall patient outcomes have improved, many centers currently include pediatric and adolescent gynecologists (PAG) in their multidisciplinary team. With such collaboration, girls can receive better care and parents can receive important counseling. Involvement by an experienced pediatric and adolescent gynecologist is a valuable investment in the provision of the best care and optimal reproductive outcomes for patients with complex genitourinary anomalies.

Associations of Genitourinary Anomalies with Reproductive Anomalies

Mullerian anomalies are known to be associated with renal anomalies in 20 percent to 40 percent cases and 30 percent of females with unilateral renal agenesis have reproductive tract anomalies [1]. Females with a known unilateral renal anomaly (including agenesis, dysgenesis, ectopic location, and dysplasia) should undergo evaluation for a concurrent reproductive tract anomaly [2]. By recognizing this association and having an increased index of suspicion, an obstructive phenomenon at menarche can be avoided. Previous reviews also support the association of Mullerian anomalies with anorectal malformations and complete evaluation of the reproductive system of such patients. In a series of 272 patients treated for imperforate anus with a rectovestibular fistula, 5 percent had an associated vaginal septum and 7 percent had an absent vagina [3]. Most pediatric surgical providers are aware of the strong association of gynecologic anomalies with a cloacal anomaly, which is cited in 53 percent to 67 percent of patients who have uterovaginal anomalies [4,5,6]. Gynecologic abnormalities seem to be relatively uncommon in patients with imperforate anus and a rectoperineal fistula. Bladder exstrophy and epispadias complex (BEEC) is usually associated with a normally developed uterus; however, that anatomic configuration of the uterus is distorted due to the angle of the interaction with the bladder. The clitoris is bifid and the vagina tends to be short (5–6 cm) and parallel to the floor when the patient is standing; the cervix is found low down, near the introitus and there may be an intriotal stenosis. The incomplete configuration of the levator ani and the pelvic floor musculature means there is an increased risk of pelvic organ (uterovaginal) prolapse (POP) [7]. Each orifice is moved anteriorly.

The primary urological consideration is the safety of the upper tracts such that all of these patients will require lifelong review and surveillance of their renal architecture and function. Fundamental principles also apply – they need a reservoir to store urine, a continence mechanism, and a means by which urine can be emptied.

In cloacal anomalies, the ability to achieve continence with spontaneous voiding relates to the length of the common channel (CC). A CC longer than 3 cm is more complex to reconstruct and less likely to have continence (i.e., dry and voiding spontaneously) than those with a shorter CC. BEEC or female epispadias involve an open urethral sphincter. Part of the early surgery will be to reconstruct this and close the bladder. Many patients (81 percent) require bladder augmentation with a cystoplasty; 70 percent will require urinary diversion – this occurs at a mean age of 11 years [8]. There are a variety of techniques for urinary diversion including vesicostomy, ureterostomy, ileal conduit (all incontinent stomas), a continent catheterizable channel (Mitrofanoff) with or without cystoplasty, and a ureterosigmoidostomy (ureters anastomosed to a sigmoid/rectal pouch with a dual fecal and urinary stream). All have both advantages and disadvantages with the need for long-term follow-up. These are complex patients and need lifelong care in a specialized center.

Understanding Reproductive Anatomy

It is essential to understand the type of reproductive anomaly and expected effects both on short- and long-term outcomes. Non-obstructive uterovaginal anomalies will not produce acute concerns either in infancy or at menarche, thus management may be deferred until later adolescence or young adulthood. Since possible menstrual obstruction at puberty may lead to catastrophic consequences, obstructive anomalies should be identified and addressed early. In cases with complex genitourinary anatomy, it is essential to fully understand the uterovaginal anatomy to prevent these adverse outcomes. Previous literature has reported a 36 percent to 41 percent rate of menstrual obstruction at puberty [9] with some complex anomalies, such as cloaca. If not diagnosed early, not only can this complication produce significant pain, often requiring urgent surgical intervention, but it can also lead to infertility. In patients with less pelvic anatomic complexity, undiagnosed obstructive phenomenon may have less profound consequences; thus, management could potentially be deferred until postpuberty. However, recent evidence suggests that families may be interested and receptive to learning of these concerns earlier [10]. If patients are undergoing early surgery of the urinary or colorectal systems, uterovaginal anomalies, such as a longitudinal non-obstructive vaginal septum, may be effectively treated in one procedure. This can be accomplished with one anesthetic exposure, with optimal surgical exposure, and without possible psychosocial concerns seen in adolescence.

The timing of an accurate assessment of reproductive anatomy is recommended before or during the definitive repair of any complex genitourinary anomaly. This can be performed preoperatively using radiologic modalities or optimally under coincident anesthesia at the time of definitive surgical repair of the anomaly. The multidisciplinary surgical team should be prepared to undertake any necessary surgical intervention such as vaginal septum resection or resection of atretic Mullerian remnants, if diagnosed. Conveniently, in many complex malformations such as BEEC or cloaca, an exam under anesthesia with both cystoscopy and vaginoscopy is often undertaken for the benefit of surgical planning. Such examination may allow definitive information about adequate outflow. Assessment of the internal reproductive anatomy may also be performed whenever an intra-abdominal procedure is performed. Since patients with complex pelvic anatomy often undergo multiple intra-abdominal procedures such as creation and takedown of a colostomy or urinary diversion procedures, these may be additional surgical opportunities to assess and document internal reproductive anatomy. However, since in many cases the reproductive anatomy was not evaluated at any of these early opportunities, this assessment can be performed later, with the combination of laparoscopy at the time of creation of an appendico-vesicostomy (a continent catheterizable channel) as indicated for bladder management. Some patient may need complex bowel management – these tend to be confined to neuropathic patients, cloacal exstrophy, and some cloacal anomalies. This may include the formation of an antegrade continent enema (ACE) channel or colostomy/ileostomy. Any reconstructive surgery may represent another opportunity for assessment. The goal is to have as much information as possible regarding reproductive anatomy so that a definitive plan can be in place for implementation on or around the onset of menarche. Accurate knowledge of the reproductive anatomy allows both parents and providers to adequately prepare well ahead of anticipated pubertal changes and arrange necessary surveillance or planned interval procedures.

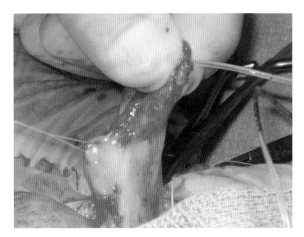

Figure 9B.1 Saline perturbation of the Fallopian tube performed during an open laparotomy during reconstructive surgery as a child to confirm patency of the reproductive tract for future menstruation.

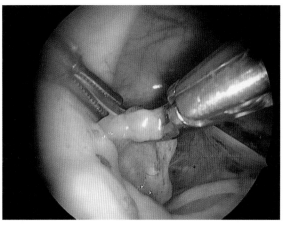

Figure 9B.2 Saline perturbation of the Fallopian tube performed during a laparoscopy for another indication prior to the onset of puberty to confirm patency of the reproductive tract for future menstruation.

During either a laparoscopy or laparotomy, the uterus/uteri should be identified and location(s) within the pelvis documented. The insertion of the Fallopian tubes into the uterine body should be recorded, in addition to the communication of the Fallopian tubes with the ovaries. Documentation of patency of the Mullerian system should also be considered. Pediatric feeding tubes can be used to cannulate the distal aspect of each Fallopian tube; gentle compression of the fimbriae around the tube allows the antegrade instillation of saline through the Fallopian tube, uterus, cervix, and vagina of the Mullerian system bilaterally (Figure 9B.1). This assessment of patency can provide reassurance regarding the future outflow of menstrual products. Initially described during open laparotomy procedures, this assessment of the Mullerian system may also be performed during laparoscopy. Antegrade instillation of saline may be performed using laparoscopic instrumentation with the same pediatric feeding tube (Figure 9B.2).

Uterovaginal Concerns Identified in Infancy

Hydrocolpos

The most significant gynecologic concern during infancy is the presence of hydrocolpos. Hydrocolpos involves the accumulation of fluid, likely urine, within the vagina causing distension of the vagina or hemivaginas. Secondary obstruction of the urinary tract can occur with the development of hydroureter and/or hydronephrosis. The definitive etiology of hydrocolpos is unclear; however, it seems to occur more commonly in females with vaginal duplication, a complex cloaca (CC; particularly in cases with a long CC), or patients with urogenital sinus anomalies (also referred to as posterior type cloaca by some expert surgeons). In the literature, the incidence of hydrocolpos in cloaca patients has been between 28 percent and 34 percent [11]. In a previous review of 645 patients with cloaca, data regarding hydrocolpos were available for 638 patients and data regarding reproductive anatomy were available for 622 patients. Uterovaginal duplication was a statistically significant association in cloaca patients with hydrocolpos [12].

The treatment of choice for persistent hydrocolpos is drainage of the vagina with vaginostomy, which can be performed with other medically indicated procedures, such as creation of a colostomy. A pigtail catheter can be placed transabdominally that should be left in place until the definitive surgical repair of the genital anomaly. Other techniques have not been shown to be effective in decreasing risk for infection, including sepsis, or persistent inflammation that may adversely affect mobilization at the definitive surgical repair [13]. If a vaginal septum is present with two hemivaginas, a window within the septum is needed to allow adequate drainage of both hemivaginas, with a single tube. When creating the window, attention should be paid to the location of the cervix on each side of the septum. Most such cervices are located very close to the septum at the superior aspect and often at the similar levels of the vagina. Trauma or damage to the cervix even in infancy has the potential to increase the risk of cervical insufficiency as an adult woman. Cervical insufficiency is a recognized cause of mid-trimester pregnancy loss [14]. Vesicostomy may be necessary in select cases, when a patient has a solitary kidney, a cloaca with an extremely long CC, or high insertion of the vagina in patients with a persistent urogenital sinus or evidence of renal insufficiency. Unification of the two hemivaginas and resection of a vaginal septum may be addressed at the definitive surgical repair for most patients undergoing complex pelvic reconstruction.

Vaginal Septum

During infancy and childhood, the presence of a longitudinal non-obstructing vaginal septum has no clinical ramifications. However, as young women enter puberty and become menarchal, they may desire to use tampons for menstrual hygiene. The presence of a vaginal septum prevents effective use of a tampon for menstrual flow and may, in adult women, cause painful vaginal intercourse. The definitive surgical repair of the urogenital anomaly may allow desirable surgical exposure and access for the opportunity to resect the distal aspect of the septum and unify the distal vagina. The advantages of resecting the septum at the definitive repair include a single anesthetic exposure, optimal surgical exposure, and the ability to effectively use tampons for menstrual hygiene beginning at menarche, if desired.

Puberty and Menarche

Ovarian function is normal in girls with complex urogenital anomalies, with the possible exception of conditions of disorders of sexual development (DSD). In DSD conditions, gonadal development may be affected, thus impacting both anatomic development of the genitalia during the fetal period and hormonal function at the time of puberty. Outside of DSD conditions, most patients are expected to have normal ovarian development and function. Thus, pubertal and breast development should occur as expected. Breast development signifies the "turning on" of the hypothalamic-pituitary-ovarian axis. Despite the earlier onset of breast and pubic hair development, the onset of menses, or menarche, has remained stable

over the past 40 years at 12.7 to 12.9 years in the United States [15,16,17]. Therefore, a window of opportunity exists to prevent the accumulation of obstructed menstrual fluid if the reproductive anatomy is not patent. Generally, the time period from the onset of breast development until menarche ranges from 1 to 3 years, which is the ideal time for evaluation. However, the timing of menarche can be affected by a number of factors, including family history, ovarian function, development of the uterine structure, and the persistence and patency of the reproductive tract. It is important to inquire about the onset of menses in all pubertal females who have undergone urogenital reconstruction, especially if a reproductive anomaly is known to be present.

Risk of Obstructive Menstruation

Effective menstruation requires adequate uterine development, with the presence of endometrium within the uterine body and a patent outflow tract. Underdeveloped structures may have variable amounts of endometrium, but if present, they require an adequate outflow tract. Confirmation of the patency of the reproductive tract before menarche has been recommended as an important technique to avoid obstruction, pain, and risk to reproductive organs and fertility. If young women reach puberty without such an assessment, clinical and ultrasound follow-up is recommended on a regular basis to follow menstrual frequency, adequacy, and possible signs or symptoms of obstruction (cyclic followed by persistent lower quadrant or pelvic pain). In young adult women, established methods, such as retrograde instillation of contrast material using fluoroscopy can provide beneficial information (hysterosalpingogram).

Parents, primary care providers, and other members of the medical team should be counseled regarding expectations and precautions. Ultrasound surveillance of the reproductive structures should be considered as an adjunct for early detection of signs of obstruction. With pelvic ultrasounds beginning about 6 to 9 months after the onset of breast development and continuing every 6 to 9 months through menarche, unexpected obstructive complications can be avoided. The actual images should be reviewed with special attention to endometrial thickness in the uterine body (bodies). If an obstruction to menstrual flow is detected by visualization of a thickened endometrium with hematometra and/or hematocolpos, hormonal suppression should be initiated immediately to minimize adverse sequelae.

Hormonal suppression of endometrial stimulation and menses prevents continued accumulation of obstructed menstrual products. It allows symptom relief and resolution of inflammatory changes, and it increases the potential for salvage of reproductive structures. After inflammatory changes have resolved and retained menstrual fluid has been drained and/or resorbed, surgery may be performed to establish an adequate outflow tract or resect atretic structures.

Patients with cloacal exstrophy may be at even greater risk of concerns at the time of puberty and menstruation. There is a well-known association of uterovaginal duplication in girls born with cloacal exstrophy [18]; however, the uteri and vaginas can be widely spaced, even at opposite sides of the separated pelvis. In this situation, it is not uncommon to fail to recognize the existence of one side of the Mullerian system at the time of definitive repair, leaving a risk of obstruction at menarche and the need for more surgery in an already tenuous abdomen and pelvis. Unilateral surgical resection of an atretic Mullerian structure may avoid future problems if a well-developed hemiuterus with a patent outflow tract is present on the opposite side. This is especially important in patients with cloacal exstrophy, as they will likely have more a complex surgical abdomen with possible bladder augmentation/neobladder, continent catherizable bladder access (Mitrofanoff), and an appendicostomy or permanent stoma for bowel management. Subsequent takedown and replacement of these continent conduits during surgery for the reproductive tract can potentially put the continence mechanism and integrity of these quality-of-life improving interventions at risk.

Other Gynecologic Issues

Other gynecologic concerns for pubertal females include the development of adnexal cysts, hydrosalpinges, endometriosis, and chronic pelvic pain. The risk of endometriosis significantly increases with an obstruction of the Mullerian system but may also be seen in patients with congenitally displaced endometrium. Chronic pelvic pain may be related to the development of endometriosis or pubertal stimulation of chronically adhesed distorted reproductive anatomy from chronic lower abdominal or pelvic adhesions.

Reproduction

Even when their daughter is only an infant, reproductive potential is already on the minds of parents. Parents are anxious to learn if their daughter will be able to have normal sexual intimacy and carry a pregnancy as an adult woman. In fact, recently presented data showed that parents who were informed of their daughter's associated gynecologic anatomy at the time of her ARM (anorectal malformation) diagnosis were more likely to report this timing as ideal. When parents were informed earlier about their daughter's associated gynecologic anomalies, they were significantly more confident in their ability to make health care decisions [10].

Sexual intimacy

Many young women who were born with complex urogenital anomalies enjoy healthy sexual relationships and may be able to become pregnant. Warne and others provided promising information in the adult cloacal reconstruction population with 12/21 (57 percent) patients reporting participation in vaginal intercourse [9]. Continued follow-up is necessary to fully appreciate the sexual outcomes in this population. Preliminary data suggest that young women with all anorectal malformations have the potential for both sexual and reproductive success [19].

In any young woman with a urogenital anomaly, a complete physical examination after puberty is necessary to evaluate secondary sexual development with the benefit of hormonal stimulation. Such an exam allows an objective determination of the adequacy of the reproductive anatomy for sexual intimacy. Examination of the introital area should be performed to assess for possible vaginal and/or introital stenosis. The perineal body should also be examined with attention to integrity/strength, presence of any scarring, and pliability. An inadequate perineal body may be problematic for sexual intimacy or spontaneous vaginal delivery of an infant.

Even if the introitus is adequate for menstrual flow, it may be inadequate for intercourse. The hormonally stimulated adult vaginal introitus should be able to accommodate at least a #26 size Hegar dilator for comfortable sexual activity. The majority of girls with BEEC undergo an early vaginoplasty with the standard posterior fourchette incision with the use of an inverted U-flap, with >20 percent requiring an introitoplasty later and 10 percent reported previous vaginal dilation

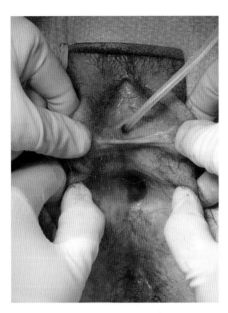

Figure 9B.3 Intraoperative views of an introitoplasty performed in late adolescence to allow comfortable sexual intimacy in a patient with a cloaca initially reconstructed during early childhood. (Preop image)

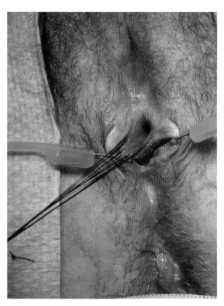

Figure 9B.4 Intraoperative views of an introitoplasty performed in late adolescence to allow comfortable sexual intimacy in a patient with a cloaca initially reconstructed during early childhood. (Intra-op image)

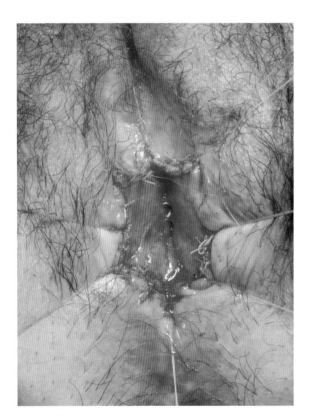

Figure 9B.5 Intraoperative views of an introitoplasty performed in late adolescence to allow comfortable sexual intimacy in a patient with a cloaca initially reconstructed during early childhood. (Completed OR image)

[20]. Many young women can perform self-dilation using vaginal dilators, or Hegar dilators, to stretch a small band of scar that may preclude comfortable sexual relations. In cases of more significant scarring, an introito/vaginoplasty may be necessary. In patients with BEEC or other urogenital anomalies, this may be an outpatient procedure in which the vaginal introitus is circumferentially mobilized to excise the scarred segment and exteriorize the soft pliable upper vagina (Figures 9B.3, 9B.4, 9B.5). Preoperatively, an assessment of the degree of stenosis, including the amount and depth of scarring and the adequacy of the perineal body, is essential. If the segment of stenosis is too thick and/or an inadequate segment of vagina exists above it, consideration of distal vaginal replacement or other augmentation grafts may be indicated. Such a procedure may require a full bowel preparation or in some circumstances may include an abdominal exploration for a bowel graft. If the perineal body is too short to accommodate a larger vaginal introitus, creative solutions may be necessary such as mobilization and expansion anteriorly especially in women who may have previously undergone bladder neck closure and creation of an abdominal catheterizable channel. Often short-term vaginal dilation, during the constrictive phase of healing, will be necessary postoperatively until adequate healing allows for vaginal intercourse.

Recent literature supports the role of buccal mucosa grafts for augmentation vaginoplasty in cases with a thickened segment of scarring or overall inadequate vagina for perineal advancement [21,22,23]. The advantages of using buccal tissue over bowel neovaginal grafts include the similarity to native vaginal mucosa, elimination of bowel prep, avoidance of an extended time without oral intake and parenteral nutrition during the postoperative recovery, and elimination of risk to adequate bowel control. Relative disadvantages include lengthy hospitalization at bed rest with urinary diversion with an indwelling Foley catheter (suprapubic catheter for patients with a persistent hypospadic urethra), subjective difficulties moving bowels while at extended bed rest (7 days), and a finite amount of obtainable graft tissue to cover needed areas of stricture. This option has provided an additional choice for patients requiring both small and large grafts as well as primary or secondary procedures. Currently, the primary role has been in pubertal patients due to the need for vaginal stenting for the entire immediate postoperative recovery followed by daily vaginal dilations beginning a few weeks after surgery.

Vaginal reconstruction is necessary in cases in which the native vagina is congenitally absent or unable to be mobilized to reach the perineum at the time of surgical reconstruction. It is always preferable to retain native vagina whenever possible; however, other tissue sources have been utilized to construct a functional vagina. Multiple authors have reported on cases of vaginal replacement using a segment of bowel to replace some or all of the native vagina [24]. Several complications were noted in the retrospective review, including mucus production, stenosis, neovaginal prolapse, and fistula formation. In our review, the most common complication was introital stenosis affecting 14 percent of all cases. Interestingly, mucus production was reported only in patients with a rectal neovaginal segment.

Pregnancy

Pregnancy is possible in women born with urogenital anomalies, even in the most complex malformations [25,26,27]. In adult women born with a congenital anomaly affecting the urethra and vagina, sparing the uterine anatomy, pregnancy rates and outcomes should be similar to the rest of the population, dependent on other medical factors, such as kidney function, as evidenced by serum creatinine levels, or blood pressure levels. Early literature noted an elevated maternal mortality rate (4 percent) for patients with BEEC; however, more recent reports suggest that rate to be more like the remaining population. Patients are at increased risk of preterm delivery, preeclampsia, and breech presentation [27]. Increased rates of pelvic organ prolaspe (POP) are notable in this population and are thought to increase with pregnancy and vaginal delivery. Deans and colleagues noted that 57 percent of women with BEEC reported POP and of these 88 percent required surgery [20]. In women with an associated reproductive anomaly (most commonly a Mullerian anomaly), the specific type of anomaly will influence the potential for conception and pregnancy risks [28,29]. Limited fertility and pregnancy data are available regarding women with a number of complex anomalies.

Recommended obstetric management begins before pregnancy with a preconceptual counseling visit with a maternal fetal medicine physician. Such consultation allows a review of previous operative procedures; determination of the known reproductive anatomy; and evaluation for concurrent medical issues, such as the development of renal insufficiency, which may influence plans for pregnancy. During pregnancy, patients should be followed, under the shared care of an obstetrician and urologist, for signs or symptoms of preterm labor and also to ensure the safety of the upper tracts and function of the reconstructed urinary tract. Uterine anomalies increase the risk for preterm labor, preterm delivery, and abnormal presentation. Decisions about mode of delivery should be addressed individually, with consideration of previous surgeries, the presence of any stomas, and technical aspects of the definitive repair. As a general recommendation, women who had a history of BEEC should be strongly considered for delivery by cesarean section (C/S) [27]. Although limited data are available regarding pregnancies and outcomes in women with a history of a cloacal repair, the default recommendation should be for C/S. Recently presented data regarding reproductive outcomes of females with ARM revealed 40 pregnancies in 25 patients, with 9 pregnancies in 7 patients with cloaca. Of those patients, all six that carried to viability were delivered by C/S [30]. These recommendations are especially important in women who may have required an extensive surgical repair for good functional outcome. Also, patients who have a neovaginal replacement or interposition graft require C/S to avoid irreparable damage to the graft. The obstetrician should consult with a pediatric or reconstructive urologist/surgeon to discuss the approach and request intraoperative consultation to protect continent conduits, such as a Mitrofanoff or appendicostomy or critical blood supply of possible augmented bladder segment. Vaginal delivery may be an option in women who underwent a more straightforward repair and have a complete native vagina. Women who do not rely upon good perineal sensation and sphincter control to be clean and dry may be candidates for spontaneous vaginal delivery. Perineal laceration causing trauma to the anal sphincter will be less likely to produce negative changes to bowel control and quality of life in women using daily enemas to remain clean and dry. Such patients are more likely to have undergone multiple abdominal surgeries with an increased chance of adhesions and possible appendicostomy at the umbilicus making cesarean section more surgically challenging and risky for negative effects on function of the appendicostomy or continence of a Mitrofanoff. Hence, good planning is essential and if a C/S is planned, it should be at/around 37 weeks and (as noted earlier) in the presence of an appropriately trained urological surgeon.

Conclusion

Knowledge of reproductive-related issues in females with a complex urogenital anomalies allows the provision of optimal medical and surgical management in infancy, childhood, and into young adulthood. Appropriate counseling for patients and families about potential reproductive concerns that may develop many years after the definitive surgical repair allows preparation and planning to preserve future fertility.

References

1. Thompson, D.P. and H.B. Lynn, Genital anomalies associated with solitary kidney. *Mayo Clin Proc*, 1966; **41**(8): 538–48.

2. Vallerie, A.M. and L.L. Breech, Update in Mullerian anomalies: diagnosis, management, and outcomes. *Curr Opin Obstet Gynecol*, 2010; **22**(5): 381–87.

3. Levitt, M.A., et al., Rectovestibular fistula–rarely recognized associated gynecologic anomalies. *J Pediatr Surg*, 2009; **44**(6): 1261–67; discussion 1267.

4. Hendren, W.H., Repair of cloacal anomalies: current techniques. *J Pediatr Surg*, 1986; **21**(12): 1159–76.

5. Peña, A., et al., Surgical management of cloacal malformations: a review of 339 patients. *J Pediatr Surg*, 2004; **39**(3): 470–79; discussion 470–79.

6. Raffensperger, J.G. and M.L. Ramenofsky, The management of a cloaca. *J Pediatr Surg*, 1973; **8**(5): 647–57.

7. Nakhal, R.S., et al., Genital prolapse in adult women with classical bladder exstrophy. *Int Urogynecol J*, 2012; **23**(9): 1201–5.

8. Gupta, A.D., et al., Examining long-term outcomes of bladder exstrophy: a 20-year follow-up. *BJU Int*, 2014; **113**(1): 137–41.

9. Warne, S.A., et al., Long-term gynecological outcome of patients with persistent cloaca. *J Urol*, 2003; **170**(4 Pt 2): 1493–96.

10. Morse, D., *Females with Anorectal Malformation (ARM): When Is the Best Time to Inform Parents/Guardians of Associated Gynecologic Anomalies?* 2015; Cincinnati Children's Hospital Medical Center.

11. Bischoff, A., et al., Hydrocolpos in cloacal malformations. *J Pediatr Surg*, 2010; **45**(6): 1241–45.

12. Chan S, S.B., Alexander M., Hossain M., Martinez-Leo B., Bischoff A., Dickie B. et al., *Association of Uterovaginal Anomalies with Hydrocolpos and Common Channel Length in Patients with Cloacal Malformations*, in *North American Society for Pediatric and Adolescent Gynecology Annual Meeting*, 2015; Orlando, FL.

13. Chalmers, D.J., et al., Clean intermittent catheterization as an initial management strategy provides for adequate preservation of renal function in newborns with persistent cloaca. *J Pediatr Urol*, 2015; **11**(4): 211 e1–4.

14. Cunningham, F., et al., *Abortion*, in *Williams Obstetrics*, F. Cunningham, et al., eds. New York: McGraw-Hill, 2001; 855–82.

15. Wu, T., P. Mendola, and G.M. Buck, Ethnic differences in the presence of secondary sex characteristics and menarche among US girls: the Third National Health and Nutrition Examination Survey, 1988–1994. *Pediatrics*, 2002; **110**(4): 752–57.

16. Chumlea, W.C., et al., Age at menarche and racial comparisons in US girls. *Pediatrics*, 2003; **111**(1): 110–13.

17. Herman-Giddens, M.E., et al., Secondary sexual characteristics and menses in young girls seen in office practice: a study from the Pediatric Research in Office Settings network. *Pediatrics*, 1997; **99**(4): 505–12.

18. Tank, E.S. and S.M. Lindenauer, Principles of management of exstrophy of the cloaca. *Am J Surg*, 1970; **119**(1): 95–98.

19. Chan S, S.B., Alexander M., Martinez-Leo B., Bischoff A., Dickie B., Frischer J. et al., *Pregnancy Outcomes in Patients with Anorectal Malformations*, in *North American Society for Pediatric and Adolescent Gynecology Annual Meeting*. 2015; Orlando, FL.

20. Deans, R., et al., Sexual function and health-related quality of life in women with classic bladder exstrophy. *BJU Int*, 2015; **115**(4): 633–38.

21. Samuelson, M.L. and L.A. Baker, *Autologous buccal mucosa vulvovaginoplasty for high urogenital sinus*. *J Pediatr Urol*, 2006; **2**(5): 486–88.

22. Oakes, M.B., et al., Augmentation vaginoplasty of colonic neovagina stricture using oral mucosa graft. *J Pediatr Adolesc Gynecol*, 2010; **23**(1): e39–42.

23. Grimsby, G.M., K. Bradshaw, and L.A. Baker, *Autologous buccal mucosa graft augmentation for foreshortened vagina*. *Obstet Gynecol*, 2014; **123**(5): 947–50.

24. Hermann, L., et al., *Bowel Vaginopolasty Associated with Complex Anorectal Malformations: A Retrospective Review of 131 Cases*. San Antonio, TX: North American Society for Pediatric & Adolescent Gynecology, 2009; e17–18.

25. Deans, R., et al., Reproductive outcomes in women with classic bladder exstrophy: an observational cross-sectional study. *Am J Obstet Gynecol*, 2012; **206**(6): 496 e1–6.

26. Dy, G.W., et al., Successful pregnancy in patients with exstrophy-epispadias complex: a University of Washington experience. *J Pediatr Urol*, 2015; **11**(4): 213 e1–6.

27. Eswara, J.R., et al., The recommendations of the 2015 American Urological Association Working Group on Genitourinary Congenitalism. *Urology*, 2016; **88**: 1–7.

28. Chan, Y.Y., et al., Reproductive outcomes in women with congenital uterine anomalies: a systematic review. *Ultrasound Obstet Gynecol*, 2011; **38**(4): 371–82.

29. Hua, M., et al., Congenital uterine anomalies and adverse pregnancy outcomes. *Am J Obstet Gynecol*, 2011; **205**(6): 558 e1–5.

30. Chan, S.H., et al., Pregnancy outcomes in patients with anorectal malformations. *Journal of Pediatric and Adolescent Gynecology*, 2015; **28**(2): e59.

Chapter 10

Late Effects of Childhood Cancer in Pediatric and Adolescent Gynecology Practice

Leslie A. Appiah and Melanie C. Davies

Introduction

Cancer affects 1 in 500 children up to the age of 14, and cancer incidence rises with age. Each year in the United States approximately 15,780 children between birth and age 19 are diagnosed with cancer. The commonest cancers occurring in childhood are leukemia, brain/CNS tumors, and lymphoma, and in teenagers, in addition to these, sarcomas of bone and soft tissue, carcinomas, germ cell tumors, and malignant melanoma. Early diagnosis and advancements in treatments have resulted in survival rates of 83 percent and 84 percent respectively for childhood (ages 0–14) and adolescent (15–19) cancer survivors [1,2]. As a result of improved therapies, it is predicted that 1 in 800 women will be childhood cancer survivors by 2020 and therefore at risk of long-term sequelae, or "late effects" of therapy. To appropriately address late effects, comprehensive care of the cancer survivor should be provided to include counseling regarding fertility preservation, contraception, and menstrual suppression prior to therapy and assessment of reproductive function, hormonal status, and sexual dysfunction in survivorship [3,4,5]. Reproductive late effects to be addressed include ovarian insufficiency and its sequelae of delayed puberty, impaired fertility, decreased bone mass, and impaired vaginal health, as well as increased risk of cardiovascular disease, early onset dementia, and Parkinson's. Sexual dysfunction is an important late effect of pelvic radiation and surgery that is often not addressed. This chapter reviews the late effects of childhood cancer in the pediatric and adolescent gynecology practice and provides evidence-based guidance to care in a problem-based approach.

Effects of Cancer Treatment

Acute ovarian failure in childhood cancer survivors has been reported at 6 percent in the Childhood Cancer Survivor Study as compared to 0.8 percent of their siblings [6]. Moreover, the risk of diminished ovarian reserve remains with the risk of imminent ovarian failure reported to be as high as 22.6 percent and the risk of premature menopause 8 percent after alkylating agent therapy, depending on the age at diagnosis [7,8]. Premature menopause is associated with sequelae of osteoporosis, early onset dementia, and morbidity and mortality related to cardiovascular disease [9,10].

The degree of ovarian injury depends on the age at therapy, treatment type, with alkylating agents being especially gonadotoxic, and total cumulative dose, with multi-dose therapies having a cumulative toxic effect on ovarian function [11](Table 10.1). Green and colleagues developed the "cyclophosphamide equivalent dose" scoring system to stratify survivors at high risk of ovarian failure. A CED $\geq$ 7.5 gm/m^2 is associated with a relative risk of premature menopause of 4.19 and may be used to counsel survivors regarding fertility preservation options [12]. It is well established that radiation doses to the ovary > 2 Gy result in a loss of 50 percent of follicles and impaired fertility [13]. Pelvic radiation doses $\geq$ 15 Gy in prepubertal and 10 Gy in postpubertal females have permanent effects on the ovary and are associated with a high risk of ovarian failure. Craniospinal radiation $\geq$ 25 Gy is associated with diminished function of the hypothalamic-pituitary axis, which can develop several years after treatment, leading to secondary ovarian insufficiency. Pelvic radiation doses $\geq$ 30 Gy are associated with irreversible injury to the uterus. Pelvic radiation and total body irradiation (TBI) result in impaired uterine growth in prepubertal children and restricted uterine blood flow with the consequences of spontaneous abortion, premature birth and low birth weight offspring [14,15].

Predicting the extent of reproductive impairment and the window of fertility for family planning has proven challenging. Assessment of ovarian reserve with anti-Müllerian hormone (AMH) and antral follicle count (AFC) is useful in predicting response and pregnancy

Table 10.1 Risk of treatment-related infertility after cancer therapies

Degree of risk	Type of therapy	Examples
High risk >80 percent risk of permanent amenorrhea in women	– HSC transplantation with cyclophosphamide/TBI or cyclophosphamide/busulfan – External beam radiation to a field that includes the ovaries	– Relapsed leukemia/lymphoma – Cervical cancer
Intermediate risk 40–60 percent risk of permanent amenorrhea in women	– BEACOPP – CMF, CEF, CAF, TAC x 6 cycles in women age 30–39	– Hodgkin's lymphoma – Breast cancer
Low risk <20 percent risk of permanent amenorrhea in women	– ALL multi-agent therapy – AML therapy (anthracycline/cytarabine) – ABVD in women ≥ 32 years – CHOP x 4–6 cycles – CMF, CEF, CAF, TAC x 6 cycles in women ≤ 30 years	– Acute lymphoblastic leukemia (first-line therapy) – Acute myeloid leukemia (first-line therapy) – Hodgkin's lymphoma – Non-Hodgkin's lymphoma – Breast cancer
Very low risk of permanent amenorrhea	– ABVD in women <32 years – Methotrexate – Tamoxifen	– Hodgkin's lymphoma – Rheumatological conditions – Breast cancer
Unknown risk	– Monoclonal antibodies – Tyrosine kinase inhibitors	– Trastuzumab for breast cancer – Imatinib for chronic myeloid leukemia

Adapted from Lambertini M, Del Mastro L, Pescio MC et al. Cancer and fertility preservation: international recommendations from an expert meeting. BMC Medicine 2016; 14:1. http://bmcmedicine.biomedcentral.com/articles/10.1186/s12916-015-0545-7

rates from assisted reproduction in infertile women; however, there is limited data on how to best use ovarian reserve markers in counseling young cancer survivors [16,17]. Nomograms to predict the age of menopause in healthy women have been reported showing that AMH and age were significantly correlated with the time to menopause and useful as predictors [18,19]. However, such nomograms have not been used to predict loss of the fertility window in survivors of childhood cancers (Figure 10.1).

Intracranial cancers (and benign tumors) may affect the hypothalamic-pituitary-ovarian (HPO) axis function due to mass effect, hormonal production, and the treatment itself. The radiation dose to the hypothalamus and pituitary that confers damage is >30 Gy of radiation. Scatter effect may also affect the hypothalamic-pituitary function. Disruption of the HPO axis results in decreased gonadotropins with resultant estrogen insufficiency. Disruption of the anterior pituitary may cause a decrease in adrenocorticotropic hormone, growth hormone, luteinizing hormone, follicle stimulating hormone, prolactin, and thyroid hormone. Disruption of the posterior pituitary results in decreased anti-diuretic hormone and oxytocin. These hormone deficiencies are typically identified and managed by pediatric endocrinologists. Pediatric gynecologists may co-manage hormone replacement therapy of survivors with estrogen insufficiency. With permanent damage to the HPO axis, estrogen replacement is required until the expected age of menopause.

Cancers of the Reproductive Tract

Cancers of the reproductive tract in childhood are rare but highly curable. They include primary ovarian, uterine, vaginal, and vulvar cancers. Secondary uterine cancers may be observed in young adulthood as a consequence of prior radiation to the pelvis. Ovarian cancers in children represent 0.2 percent of all ovarian neoplasms with germ cell tumors accounting for 70 percent of ovarian tumors in children [20]. Sex cord stromal tumors are the second most common childhood ovarian malignancy followed by epithelial tumors, which represent 7 percent of ovarian malignancies in children. Fertility-sparing surgery with unilateral oophorectomy is recommended for low-grade ovarian malignancies. Combination chemotherapy with bleomycin, etoposide, and cisplatin (BEP) or carboplatin is reserved for higher-grade ovarian cancers. Cancers of the uterus, vagina, and vulva are often rhabdomyosarcomas. Treatment

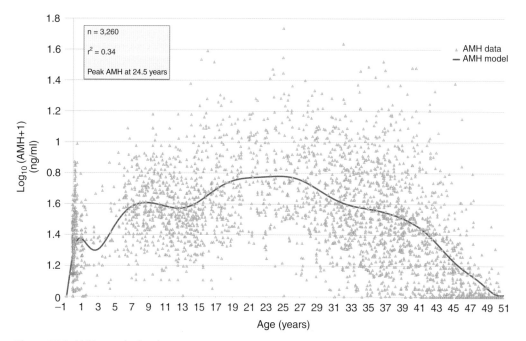

Figure 10.1 AMH normal values by age
Kelsey TW, Wright P, Nelson SM, Anderson RA, Wallace WH. A validated model of serum anti-Müllerian hormone from conception to menopause.
http://journals.plos.org/plosone/article?id=10.1371/journal.pone.0022024

regimens include surgery, chemotherapy, and radio-therapy (brachytherapy and/or external beam irradiation) with 5-year survival rates >90 percent [21]. Long-term complications of intensive therapy include genitourinary or digestive disorders and sexual dysfunction. The most common vaginal complaints are vaginal dryness and dyspareunia from stenosis and fibrosis [22,23]. Toxicities may last for 8–10 years based on the type of malignancy and treatment regimen. Implementation of standard surveys during and at the end of treatment allows identification of these concerns with the ability for referral to specialists in sexual health and pelvic floor physical therapy [24].

Fertility Preservation

Professional bodies (including the American Society of Clinical Oncology, American Society for Reproductive Medicine, Canadian Fertility and Andrology Society, and the Royal Colleges in the UK) recommend fertility preservation (FP) counseling prior to initiating cancer treatment in order to provide all available options to survivors [25,26,27,28]. Standard options include oocyte, embryo, and sperm freezing for adult females

and males, respectively [29]. Oocyte and sperm freezing in adolescents requires knowledgeable discussions between the patient, parent, oncologist, and reproductive specialist. Oocyte freezing in adolescent girls is not standard care but may be performed at specialized centers [30]. Sperm freezing in adolescent boys may be challenging depending on the degree of sexual maturity and may require invasive techniques to procure sperm such as testicular aspiration under anesthesia [31]. Testicular and ovarian tissue freezing in prepubertal children is an investigational option performed under research protocols for pediatric patients at high risk of infertility [32]. There are ethical considerations in undertaking procedures that are not of immediate therapeutic value in young patients who may not have a full understanding of the future implications.

Pregnancies following regrafting of frozen-thawed ovarian tissue have been reported worldwide, making this a viable option for adolescent and adult patients who decline standard therapies or cannot delay cancer treatment to pursue those options [33,34,35,36]. Laparoscopy carries the risks of a surgical procedure. In prepubertal girls, this is the only FP option, but outcomes are still unknown.

Ovarian transposition or oophoropexy may be considered for individual cases to move the ovaries out of the field of localized radiation. Subsequently a second laparoscopy may be performed to release them and allow natural conception, or IVF may be required with egg pickup from the transposed ovary [37].

Despite our knowledge of FP options, only a minority of adult patients undertake FP therapies. Unfortunately, discussions simply may not occur, due to physicians' lack of awareness about options and concerns for treatment delay and cost of therapies [38]. At the time of diagnosis, patients receive a great amount of information. Many patients do not "hear" or are unable to process discussions about future fertility at that time. For these reasons, after an initial discussion by the oncologist, a separate conversation with a reproductive specialist is recommended. In fact, women counseled about their risk of infertility by both an oncologist and a fertility specialist had significantly less regret about their decision to preserve fertility than those counseled only by an oncologist [39].

Decision aids may assist the patient in deciding on the best option; however, few standard aids currently exist [40]. The optimal timing for discussion is prior to chemotherapy and radiation, as early referral has been reported to decrease decisional conflict by allowing time to pursue options if desired [41]. Additionally, studies suggests that adolescents desire to be a part of the decision-making process [42]. There are fewer options available once cancer treatments have started. For those patients at high risk of ovarian failure who have undergone one cycle of chemotherapy, ovarian tissue freezing remains an option. Additionally, recent studies have shown that Goserelin, a gonadotropin-releasing hormone agonist, improves pregnancy rates and long-term survival rates in patients with certain types of breast cancer [43]. Unfortunately, Goserelin has not been confirmed as an ovarian protection agent during treatment of other cancer types.

Many patients express concern that pursuing fertility options may delay cancer treatment. Ovarian stimulation for oocyte and embryo freezing require a minimum of 2 weeks. Historically, the onset of menses was required prior to initiating therapy. However, newer ovarian stimulation protocols have been developed to "quick start" stimulation during any phase of the menstrual cycle, minimizing treatment delays. Ovarian tissue freezing can be combined with cancer-related procedures and results in no delay. To optimize time to cancer therapies, FP counseling and development of a "fertility road map" should occur within days of the cancer diagnosis so that FP options can be implemented in a timely fashion. Specialist nurses to help families navigate the process, assist with financial considerations, and minimize barriers are becoming a standard and integral part of treatment teams.

Menstrual Suppression

Menstrual suppression during chemotherapy is not necessary for all cancers. However, patients receiving myeloablative agents are more likely to experience bleeding secondary to thrombocytopenia that may require transfusion and blood products; therefore, they may be candidates for menstrual suppression [44].

Menstrual suppression may be achieved in several ways. Combined oral contraceptives carry a theoretical risk of thrombosis; therefore, progestin-only options may be better. Progestin-only contraceptive pills may result in breakthrough bleeding if not taken at the same time each day. Higher doses of progestin to achieve amenorrhea may result in side effects, and in the case of norethindrone acetate, paradoxical breakthrough bleeding as estradiol is a metabolite of norethindrone acetate. Episodes of nausea and emesis during chemotherapy make oral therapy less than ideal for many patients.

Injectable medroxyprogesterone may result in breakthrough bleeding during the first 3 months. This may be difficult to control and may require additional oral progestin therapy. Additionally, an intramuscular injection in the setting of thrombocytopenia may cause hematoma formation. The dual benefit of IM medroxyprogesterone for menstrual suppression is contraception. Gonadotropin-releasing hormone agonist (GnRHa) therapy during chemotherapy downregulates the HPO axis after the initial release of gonadotropins, resulting in suppressed estradiol levels and amenorrhea. A withdrawal bleed typically occurs within 2 weeks of administration; to minimize bleeding, the ideal time to give GnRHa is during the luteal phase of the menstrual cycle or after 2 weeks of suppression with oral progestins. Unfortunately, due to the urgency surrounding initiation of chemotherapy, neither of these regimens may be ideal. Concurrent administration of oral progestin with initiation of

GnRHa therapy may be the best option. Continuing hormonal add-back therapy is advisable with prolonged administration of GnRHa therapy to minimize loss of bone mineral density [45]. Add-back therapy may be given in the form of progestin, transdermal estradiol, conjugated equine estrogen, and combined low-dose oral contraceptives. The drawbacks with estrogen therapy are breakthrough bleeding and in the case of oral contraceptives, potential for thrombosis.

Contraception

Contraception in sexually active adolescent girls is an important part of reproductive care of the patient with cancer. Pregnancy while undergoing chemotherapy or radiation treatment carries the risk of birth defects, spontaneous abortion, and iatrogenic preterm delivery. The full range of contraceptive methods is available, but contra-indications may exist to some forms of female contraception. Many patients will be at risk of thrombosis and some at very high risk, for example, during pelvic surgery or parenteral nutrition, and should avoid estrogen-containing contraceptives (the combined oral contraceptive pill, contraceptive patch and ring). Progestin contraceptives are usually preferable (the progestin-only pill, etonogestrel implantable rod, injectable medroxyprogesterone acetate), though the progestin-only pill is low dose with an increased incidence of breakthrough bleeding, particularly with missed pills; injectable medroxyprogesterone acetate and the etonogestrel implantable rod have high contraceptive efficacy but may result in initial breakthrough bleeding. The intrauterine devices have not been shown to be associated with a higher risk of infection in immunocompromised patients receiving chemotherapy. They are also approved as first-line contraceptives in sexually active adolescents [46]. The 5-year levonorgestrel intrauterine device has the highest incidence of amenorrhea of 20 percent at 1 year and 70 percent at 2 years. The 3-year levonorgestrel intrauterine device typically results in monthly bleeding. The 10-year copper IUD typically results in monthly and oftentimes heavy bleeding for the first 3 months with monthly menses thereafter.

During recovery from chemotherapy, it is important to inform young patients that even if they have amenorrhea their fertility may return, as the first ovulation occurs prior to menstruation. Contraception needs to be continued during early follow-up while there is a risk of disease recurrence.

Cancer Survivorship

Ovarian Function

Ovarian insufficiency is a concern after cancer treatment. Identifying patients at risk and developing a long-term plan to monitor gonadal function are important aspects of cancer survivorship. The menstrual cycle, while confirming ongoing ovarian activity, is not an adequate predictor of long-term fertility. Regular menses are indicative of ovulation but do not provide a window into the expected duration of fertility to attempt conception. There is currently no gold standard for monitoring fertility after treatment, however AMH and antral follicle count are currently the best available surrogate markers of ovarian reserve (Figure 10.2). Although these predict response to ovulation-induction medications, validated in IVF practice, they are unable to predict pregnancy and livebirth rates. Young patients may conceive spontaneously even with very low ovarian reserve, infrequent periods, or undetectable AMH. Routine follow-up with a reproductive specialist can help determine the best approach. For those patients who have diminished ovarian or testicular function, FP after therapy may be warranted.

It is typically recommended that patients wait until the risk of cancer recurrence is low before proceeding with pregnancy. Patients should be reassured that there is no additional risk of birth defects or miscarriages after completing chemotherapy, once cleared to attempt conception.

Induction of Puberty and HRT

Delayed puberty is a concern in patients who received highly gonadotoxic therapy prior to or during puberty. Childhood cancer survivors who are at risk for ovarian insufficiency should be followed with regular monitoring of growth and pubertal development. The Children's Oncology Group (COG) Long Term Follow-up guidelines recommend baseline assessment of FSH, LH, and estradiol at age 13, two standard deviations from the expected age of thelarche [3]. The guidelines also recommend testing when clinically indicated in patients with delayed or arrested puberty, irregular menses, primary or secondary amenorrhea, or clinical signs and symptoms of estrogen deficiency.

It is important to note that patients who receive intracranial radiation without gonadotoxic chemotherapy will have normal ovarian function although the

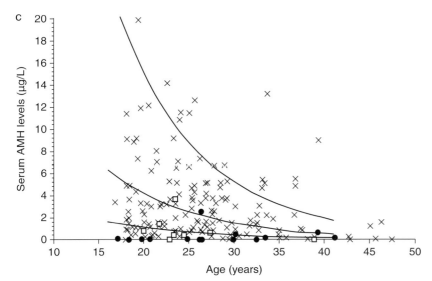

Figure 10.2 AMH after cancer therapy

Fong SL, Laven JSE, Hakvoort-Cammel FGAJ, Schipper I, Visser JA, Themmen APN et al. Assessment of ovarian reserve in adult childhood cancer survivors using anti-Müllerian hormone. *Hum. Reprod.* (2009) 24 (4): 982–90. doi: 10.1093/humrep/den487.

HPO axis is disrupted, leading to low gonadotropin and sex steroid levels. These patients will require hormone replacement therapy if they have completed puberty and estrogen replacement for pubertal induction if they have not. When they elect to conceive, they will need ovarian stimulation with gonadotropins.

There are few guidelines for induction of puberty in patients with ovarian insufficiency secondary to gonadotoxic therapy [47]. HRT is administered similarly to that of patients with Turner's syndrome [48]. The recommendations for those patients are to start off at low doses, increased every 3–6 months to achieve an adult dose of 0.1 mg/24 hour of the estradiol patch, 1–2 mg oral estradiol or 0.625 mg of conjugated equine estrogen. The goal is to mimic the natural progression of puberty. Increasing estrogen doses too rapidly will result in tubular breast formation. Progestin therapy is added after 2 years with satisfactory breast development and adequate uterine growth on ultrasound scan, or with onset of bleeding, again, similar to the natural hormonal production during puberty.

There are several regimens for HRT. Progestin-withdrawal bleeding is required to protect the uterus. The combined oral contraceptive pill, patch, and ring are convenient preparations for young women and protect against pregnancy. However, these therapies are not recommended as first-line therapies for HRT; ethinylestradiol does not provide good bioavailability to the bones and physiological replacement using estradiol provides better bone and cardiovascular protection [49]. It is important to remember that in patients with idiopathic primary ovarian insufficiency, spontaneous ovulation occurs in 25 percent of those patients, and pregnancies in 5 percent, so contraception is warranted. To maintain good bone protection, protect uterine health and contracept, a combination of estradiol with the mini-pill or levonorgestrel IUD may provide the best option. The progestin implant in combination with HRT may result in increased breakthrough bleeding. There are very few contraindications to HRT, which has not been proven to increase the risk of blood clots when given transdermally; with this route, there is no first-pass effect to increase the liver enzymes involved in clotting.

Women with premature menopause have a higher risk of early onset dementia, Parkinson's disease, and cardiac disease, and estrogen replacement may have a protective role. Low estrogen levels also result in atrophic vaginitis and dyspareunia. Patients are also susceptible to urinary tract infections, bacterial vaginosis, and vaginal candidiasis. Topical estrogen may be prescribed in addition to systemic HRT.

Sexual Dysfunction

Sexual difficulties are often overlooked as a late effect of therapy in childhood cancer survivors. As the average age of sexual debut in the United States and Europe is 17, it is important to counsel patients about this aspect of their sexuality, particularly as young women with estrogen insufficiency and those who have received pelvic radiation may experiences loss of vulvar architecture and vaginal dryness and atrophy that may result in catastrophic tearing during intercourse. Graft-versus-host disease can affect the vagina causing ulceration. Sexual dysfunction can be assessed with validated questionnaires such as the Short Sexual Functioning Scale, Specific Sexual Problems Questionnaire, and Arizona Sexual Experiences Scale. Treatment may involve topical estrogen, vaginal dilation, and in cases of graft-versus-host disease, topical steroids or tacrolimus may be given in specialist care. Referral to cognitive therapists who specialize in sexual dysfunction may be recommended. Physical therapists are also able to help with pelvic floor massage and biofeedback. A referral to a female pelvic reconstructive surgeon may be necessary to treat scarring following pelvic radiation.

Pregnancy Planning

Collaboration with a maternal fetal specialist to discuss the safety of pregnancy in the setting of certain conditions is very important. Patients who have received cardiotoxic or nephrotoxic chemotherapy should be screened prior to pregnancy. Patients with cardiac, pulmonary, and renal disease are at significant risk of peri-partum cardiomyopathy, oxygenation problems, hypertensive disorders, and thrombosis. Conception using donor oocytes also carries increased risk of pregnancy complications. Pregnancies following pelvic irradiation (including total body irradiation) are particularly high risk.

Conclusion: Key Elements for Reproductive Care of Childhood Cancer Patients

A comprehensive care program must take into account all aspects of gynecological and reproductive health care. This includes fertility preservation prior to chemotherapy, during chemotherapy, and in survivorship. It must also include sexual health. Management of long-term consequences of treatment will focus on treatment of ovarian insufficiency. Collaboration with all specialists involved in care will give the best outcomes. In survivorship, these young women may leave the care of the oncologist but will need continued health surveillance, particularly by reproductive physicians, and access to fertility specialists. Evaluation by maternal-fetal medicine at the desired time of conception is critical.

References

1. Cancer Research UK, available from www .cancerresearchuk.org/health-professional/cancer -statistics.

2. American Cancer Society. *Cancer Treatment & Survivorship Facts & Figures 2016–2017*. 2016.

3. Children's Oncology Group. *Long-term follow-up guidelines for survivors of childhood, adolescent and young adult cancers*. 2014; Version 4.0, available from: www.survivorshipguidelines.org.

4. Scottish Intercollegiate Guidelines Network. *Long term follow up of survivors of childhood cancer [SIGN132]*. 2013.

5. Lee, S.J., Schover, L.R., Partridge, A.H. et al. *American Society of Clinical Oncology recommendations on fertility preservation in cancer patients. J Clin Oncol*, 2006; **24**(18): 2917–31.

6. Chemaitilly, W., Mertens, A.C., Mitby, P. et al. *Acute ovarian failure in the childhood cancer survivor study. Journal of Clinical Endocrinology & Metabolism*, 2006; **91**(5): 1723–28.

7. Sklar, C.A., Mertens, A.C., Mitby, P. et al. *Premature menopause in survivors of childhood cancer: a report from the childhood cancer survivor study. Journal of the National Cancer Institute*, 2006; **98**(13): 890–96.

8. Lantinga, G.M., Simons, A.H., Kamps, W.A. et al. *Imminent ovarian failure in childhood cancer survivors. Eur J Cancer*, 2006; **42**(10): 1415–20.

9. Rocca, W.A., Grossardt, B.R., Shuster, L.T. *Oophorectomy, estrogen, and dementia: a 2014 update. Mol Cell Endocrinol*, 2014; **389**(1–2): 7–12.

10. Shuster, L.T., Rhodes, D. J., Gostout B.S. et al., *Premature menopause or early menopause: long-term health consequences. Maturitas*, 2010; **65**(2): 161–66.

11. Wallace, W.H.B., Anderson, R.A., Irvine, D.A. *Fertility preservation for young patients with cancer. Who is at risk and what can be offered? Lancet Oncology*, 2005; **6**(12): 922.

12. Green DM, Nolan VG, Goodman, PJ, Whitton JA, Srivastava D, Leisenring WM, et al. The cyclophosphamide equivalent dose as an approach for quantifying alkylating agent exposure: *a report from the Childhood Cancer Survivor Study. Pediatr Blood Cancer*, 2014; **61**(1): 53–67.

13. Nakayama, K., et al., *Gonadal failure after treatment of hematologic malignancies: from recognition to management for health-care providers. Nat Clin Pract Oncol*, 2008; **5**(2): 78–89.

14. Wallace, W.H.B., et al., *Predicting age of ovarian failure after radiation to a field that includes the ovaries. International Journal of Radiation Oncology Biology Physics*, 2005; **62**(3): 738–44.

15. Gao, W., Liang, J.X., Yan, Q. *Exposure to radiation therapy is associated with female reproductive health among childhood cancer survivors: a meta-analysis study. J Assist Reprod Genet*, 2015; **32**(8): 1179–86.

16. Larsen EC, Muller J, Rechnitzer C, Schmiegelow K and Andersen AN. Diminished ovarian reserve in female childhood cancer survivors with regular menstrual cycles and basal FSH <10 IU/I. *Human Reproduction*, 2003; **18**: 417–22.

17. Lukaszuk, K., et al., *Anti-Mullerian hormone (AMH) is a strong predictor of live birth in women undergoing assisted reproductive technology. Reprod Biol*, 2014; **14**(3): 176–81.

18. Broer, S.L., Eijkemans M.J., Scheffer G.J. et al., *Anti-mullerian hormone predicts menopause: a long-term follow-up study in normoovulatory women. J Clin Endocrinol Metab*, 2011; **96**(8): 2532–39.

19. Tehrani, F.R., Shakeri N., Solaymani-Dodaran, M. et al., *Predicting age at menopause from serum antimullerian hormone concentration. Menopause*, 2011; **18**(7): 766–70.

20. Benson, R.C., *Ovarian tumors in childhood and adolescence. Postgrad Med*, 1971; **50**(5): 230–35.

21. Magne, N., Haie-Meder, C. *Brachytherapy for genital-tract rhabdomyosarcomas in girls: technical aspects, reports, and perspectives. Lancet Oncol*, 2007; **8**(8): 725–29.

22. Gerbaulet, A.P., et al., *Conservative treatment for lower gynecological tract malignancies in children and adolescents: the Institut Gustave-Roussy experience. Int J Radiat Oncol Biol Phys*, 1989; **17**(3): 655–58.

23. Flamant, F., et al., *Long-term sequelae of conservative treatment by surgery, brachytherapy, and chemotherapy for vulval and vaginal rhabdomyosarcoma in children. J Clin Oncol*, 1990; **8**(11): 1847–53.

24. Levy, A., et al., *Late toxicity of brachytherapy after female genital tract tumors treated during childhood: prospective evaluation with a long-term follow-up. Radiother Oncol*, 2015; **117**(2): 206–12.

25. Loren, A.W., et al., *Fertility preservation for patients with cancer: American Society of Clinical Oncology clinical practice guideline update. J Clin Oncol*, 2013; **31**(19): 2500–10.

26. Ethics Committee of the American Society for Reproductive Medicine. Fertility preservation and reproduction in patients facing gonadotoxic therapies: a committee opinion. *Fertil Steril*, 2013; **100**: 1224–31.

27. Royal College of Obstetricians and Gynaecologists, Royal College of Physicians, and Royal College of Radiologists. *Effects of cancer treatment on reproductive functions*, 2007.

28. Canadian Fertility and Andrology Society. *Fertility Preservation In Reproductive Age Woman Facing Gonadotoxic Treatments*, 2014.

29. Practice Committee of American Society for Reproductive Medicine. *Fertility preservation in patients undergoing gonadotoxic therapy or gonadectomy: a committee opinion. Fertil Steril*, 2013; **100**(5): 1214–23.

30. Oktay, K., Bedoschi, G. *Oocyte cryopreservation for fertility preservation in postpubertal female children at risk for premature ovarian failure due to accelerated follicle loss in Turner syndrome or cancer treatments. J Pediatr Adolesc Gynecol*, 2014; **27**(6): 342–46.

31. Bahadur, G., Spoudeas H.A., Davies M.C., Ralph D. *Factors affecting sperm banking for adolescent cancer patients. Archives of Disease in Childhood* 2006; **91**: 715–16.

32. Babayev, S.N. et al., *Evaluation of ovarian and testicular tissue cryopreservation in children undergoing gonadotoxic therapies. Journal of Assisted Reproduction and Genetics*, 2013; **30**(1): 3–9.

33. Donnez, J., et al., *Restoration of ovarian activity and pregnancy after transplantation of cryopreserved ovarian tissue: a review of 60 cases of reimplantation. Fertil Steril*, 2013; **99**(6): 1503–13.

34. Meirow, D., Ra'anani, H., Biderman, H. *Ovarian tissue cryopreservation and transplantation: a realistic, effective technology for fertility preservation. Methods Mol Biol*, 2014; **1154**: 455–73.

35. Demeestere, I., et al., *Live birth after autograft of ovarian tissue cryopreserved during childhood. Hum Reprod*, 2015; **30**(9): 2107–9.

36. Jensen, A.K. et al., *Outcomes of transplantations of cryopreserved ovarian tissue to 41 women in Denmark. Hum Reprod*, 2015; **30**(12): 2838–45.

37. Irtan, S., Orbach, D., Helfre, S., Sarnacki, S. *Ovarian transposition in prepubescent and adolescent girls with cancer. Lancet Oncol*, 2013; **14**(13): e601–8.

38. Quinn, G.P., Vadaparampil, S.T., Lee, J.H. et al., *Physician referral for fertility preservation in oncology patients: a national study of practice behaviors. J Clin Oncol*, 2009; **27**(35): 5952–57.

39. Niemasik, E.E., et al., *Patient perceptions of reproductive health counseling at the time of cancer diagnosis: a qualitative study of female California cancer survivors. J Cancer Surviv*, 2012; **6**(3): 324–32.

40. Ehrbar, V., et al., *Decision-making about fertility preservation-qualitative data on young cancer patients' attitudes and needs. Arch Womens Ment Health*, 2016; **19**(4): 695–99.

41. Kim, J., Mersereau, J.E. *Early referral makes the decision-making about fertility preservation easier: a pilot survey study of young female cancer survivors. Support Care Cancer*, 2015; **23**(6): 1663–67.

42. Quinn, G.P., et al., *Who decides? Decision making and fertility preservation in teens with cancer: a review of the literature. J Adolesc Health*, 2011; **49**(4): 337–46.

43. Moore, H.C., et al., *Goserelin for ovarian protection during breast-cancer adjuvant chemotherapy. N Engl J Med*, 2015; **372**(10): 923–32.

44. Bates, J.S., Buie, L.W., Woodis, C.B. *Management of menorrhagia associated with chemotherapy-induced thrombocytopenia in women with hematologic malignancy. Pharmacotherapy*, 2011; **31**(11): 1092–110.

45. DiVasta, A.D., Laufer, M.R., Gordon C.M. *Bone density in adolescents treated with a GnRH agonist and add-back therapy for endometriosis. Journal of Pediatric and Adolescent Gynecology*, 2007; **20**(5): 293–97.

46. American College of Obstetricians and Gynecologists. ACOG Committee Opinion no. 450. *Increasing use of contraceptive implants and intrauterine devices to reduce unintended pregnancy. Obstet Gynecol*, 2009; **114**(6): 1434–38.

47. Webber L, Davies M, Anderson R, Bartlett J, Braat D, Cartwright B et al. *ESHRE guideline: management of women with premature ovarian insufficiency. Human Reproduction* 2016; **31**(5): 926–37.

48. Bondy, C.A., Turner Syndrome Study Group. *Care of girls and women with Turner syndrome: a guideline of the Turner Syndrome Study Group. J Clin Endocrinol Metab*, 2007; **92**(1): 10–25.

49. Crofton PM, Evans N, Bath LE, Warner P, Whitehead TJ, Critchley HOD et al. *Physiological versus standard sex steroid replacement in young women with premature ovarian failure: effects on bone mass acquisition and turnover. Clinical Endocrinology* 2010; **73**(6): 707–714.

Laparoscopic Surgery in Pediatric and Adolescent Gynecology Practice

Thomas R. Aust, Sari L. Kives, and Alfred Cutner

Planning, Theater Setup, and Equipment

Introduction

Laparoscopic surgery is open surgery carried out through small incisions with enhanced magnification of the operative field. The advantages of a laparoscopic (or key hole) approach to the abdomen and pelvis have been well documented across the spectrum of surgical disciplines [1]. These include a significant reduction in postoperative pain, length of stay, recovery time, and adhesion formation. In children or adolescents, this will result in a faster return to school and normal activities. Laparoscopic incisions are smaller than a transverse incision and indeed a midline laparotomy. This reduction in wound visibility is especially important in children and adolescents who otherwise may be asked by contemporaries or a new partner about the reasons behind the scar. This will be especially distressing while coming to terms with the psychological impact of the diagnosis of an XY karyotype or an absent uterus.

The enhanced visualization of laparoscopic surgery is due to the greater magnification and ability to see deep into the pelvis, compared to open surgery. This is especially important in cases of Mullerian anomalies or endometriosis when the anatomy is distorted and access to the operative site is difficult to achieve.

The advantages of laparoscopic surgery for both the patient and the surgeon would indicate that this approach should be the technique of choice when operating within the abdomen and pelvis in pediatric and adolescent gynecology.

Who Should Perform These Operations and in Which Location?

The makeup of the team will depend on the age and maturity of the patient and the presenting condition.

For example a 16-year-old with an ovarian cyst can be managed in a similar manner to a young adult in terms of anesthetic and operative techniques. Conversely, a 12-year-old with a complex Mullerian anomaly may require a pediatric anesthetist, pediatric urologist, pediatric surgeon, counseling services, and an endocrinologist. In addition, the hospital environment for surgical recovery is important and needs to take into account the age of the patient and the potential need for parental support. A room covered in cartoon characters with lights-off at 7p.m. will put a young child at ease but will leave a teenager distinctly unimpressed. However, in most units adolescents are not treated on adult wards, as this is not an appropriate environment.

A team approach to surgery is paramount to optimize outcome. The requirements for the surgical team are that the correct knowledge and skills are available during the operation. These can be within the same person or more commonly across two specialties. Some of the laparoscopic surgery will be complex, and it is unlikely that an expert pediatric and adolescent gynecology (PAG) consultant who deals with all other aspects of patient management will have a sufficient laparoscopic workload to enable adequate skill acquisition. Likewise an expert laparoscopic surgeon who carries a heavy surgical workload is unlikely to have sufficient knowledge surrounding all the other aspects of care. Thus, a team approach with a PAG specialist (with the correct knowledge) operating with an adult laparoscopic specialist with the skills of dissection of the pouch of Douglas, uterovesical fold, and pelvic sidewall and proficiency in laparoscopic suturing will optimize the surgical outcome. This approach is common in units offering complex surgery to this group of patients in the UK. We would encourage anyone endeavoring to perform complex laparoscopy in the PAG setting to foster this working relationship.

Planning Surgery

The preoperative assessment in making the diagnosis and determining the indications for surgery is dealt with in the relevant chapters in this book. Likewise, consent for surgery in children and adolescents has already been covered in previous chapters. In this section, we address those aspects specifically relevant to the surgery itself.

The suitability for laparoscopic surgery needs to take into account the specifics related to the surgery itself and also general considerations. Cardiovascular reserve to enable the raised intra-abdominal pressure and head down position during surgery is not normally a concern in the younger age group. Previous abdominal surgery and the size of the patient may determine the method for obtaining a pneumoperitoneum. Previous abdominal surgery increases the risks of adhesions and hence organ damage during primary port insertion.

The requirement to use a uterine manipulator should be discussed with the patient and her family during the preoperative period, especially with girls who have never been sexually active. This may have significant social and religious implications, as there is a risk that the hymen may tear. Vaginal examination during the procedure is obviously of less significance during vaginal reconstructive procedures.

In procedures where there is a Mullerian anomaly, preoperative knowledge of the renal tract is essential as it is important to know whether there is an absent kidney or a duplex system. This information will be required during surgical dissection of the pelvic side wall. In patients with XY gonadal dysgenesis, preoperative MRI will in most cases locate the site of the gonads and hence enable preoperative planning of the surgical approach and potential requirements of a pediatric urologist where groin dissection may be required.

Theatre Setup

Surgery requires an effective team with each member having a specific role. The familiarity of the anesthetic, scrub, and circulating staff with one another, with their equipment, and with the procedures being performed will have a direct effect on the smooth running of each case.

The theater environment has to be fit for purpose. Advanced laparoscopic theatre setups will reduce stress in the operating theater and minimize risks to staff and patients [2,3]. The layout of equipment in the operating room has taken on more relevance as the technology available to the laparoscopic surgeon has increased. When open surgery was the norm, a single diathermy machine and a suction bottle were the only devices that needed to be near the operating table. With laparoscopy that has increased to include newer energy machines such as ultracision and advanced bipolar, insufflator stacks, suction/irrigation setups and multiple high-definition monitors and control screens. The layout needs to facilitate flow of equipment to the operating table without obscuring the surgeons' view of the monitors, ideally without cables running along the floor, which could represent a trip hazard in the low-light conditions of a laparoscopic theater. Having an integrated system that allows the surgeon to control gas flow, light intensity, and the recording of images rather than requesting circulating staff to do so saves time and improves efficiency.

State of the art theaters result in a quietly flowing environment in which staff feels less stressed, which allows the team to concentrate on the operation itself. This results in a more efficient and relaxed surgical environment, which enables more complex surgery to be carried out in a safer manner.

Laparoscopic Techniques and Equipment

Most laparoscopic pelvic procedures are performed in the Lloyd-Davies position to enable access to the vagina if required. Prior to insufflation, an indwelling catheter normally empties the bladder. At the end of the procedure, this can be removed if the operation was only minor. Consideration should be given to leaving the catheter overnight as trying to catheterize a child who goes into urinary retention postoperatively can be traumatic. If the uterus is present and the operation involves inspection of the pouch of Douglas or uterine manipulation, then the uterus is instrumented.

Three main methods are utilized to obtain a pneumoperitoneum: insertion of a Verres needle at the umbilicus, open entry (Hasson), and subcostal insertion of the Verres needle (Palmer's entry). Many patients in this age group will be more susceptible to vascular injury from a standard umbilical verres technique due to the short distance from the umbilicus to the major abdominal blood vessels. To minimize the risk of vascular injury, a Hasson entry technique should be considered [4].

Umbilical entry is not suitable, whether via a closed or open technique, where there is an increased risk of adhesions under the umbilicus. An alternative entry site should be used. A Verres needle or a direct optical entry at Palmers point (left upper quadrant 2 cm below the costal margin) provides a relatively safe entry into the abdomen, allowing the inside of the umbilicus to be inspected and a port placed if free of adhesions [5]. Where a subcostal entry point is utilized, there is an increased risk of damaging the stomach if it is distended. An oro-pharyngeal tube should be placed at the start of the operation [6].

Instrumentation would largely reflect the same used in adult surgery. Minimizing the number and size or the ports should be considered to enhance the cosmetic result. However, this should not be at the expense of safe efficient surgery. For most operations we utilize an umbilical 5 or 10 mm port for the laparoscope and 2 lateral ports in line with the umbilicus and very lateral. This enables good triangulation during surgery. For complex cases, we also insert a suprapubic 5 or 10 mm port to enable additional manipulation by the assistant. In cases where further ports to enable retraction would be useful, we insert needles to carry this out without the need for ports [7].

Laparoscopic Management of Benign Ovarian Masses and Endometriosis

General Considerations

The first consideration when deciding on surgical treatment of a presumed benign ovarian mass is preservation of ovarian function. An ovarian cystectomy is always preferred over an oophorectomy as many follicles are left behind after cystectomy and can serve as oocytes for reproduction in the future. The amount of tissue remaining from the ovary after a cystectomy can also alter future fertility.

Among adolescents, the most common benign ovarian masses are functional cysts and benign neoplasms. There is a bimodal distribution of functional cysts, peaking during the fetal/neonatal and perimenarchal ages. As these cysts are usually benign and resolve spontaneously, every effort should be made to manage them expectantly with serial ultrasound prior to considering surgery.

Paratubal and paraovarian cysts may mimic simple ovarian cysts in both presentation and imaging. Surgical management is usually suggested for any adnexal cyst greater than 4 cm that fails to regress. Surgical intervention will prevent potential torsion as well as provide a pathologic diagnosis. Fortunately, the majority of ovarian cysts can be managed by laparoscopy.

Neoplastic ovarian masses in the pediatric and adolescent population include tumors of germ cell, epithelial, sex cord stromal, and metastatic of other origins. Germ cell tumors are the most common histological subtype in adolescents. Because non epithelial masses predominate in the adolescent, the following discussion focuses on the most common benign germ cell tumor, the mature cystic teratoma.

Dermoid Cysts

Mature cystic teratomas, or dermoid cysts, arise from ectodermal, mesodermal, and endodermal tissue and are the most common benign ovarian tumor found in children and adolescents. The majority of surgeons agree that symptomatic, large, and atypical dermoids require surgical removal. In asymptomatic patients, the age of the patient, future fertility, and cyst size are considered when deciding if surgery is indicated.

Traditionally, dermoid ovarian cysts have been removed by laparotomy. More recently, surgeons prefer a laparoscopic approach for treating ovarian cysts, as it is associated with less blood loss, shorter hospital stay, and fewer intraoperative and postoperative complications.

Normally, a three-port technique will suffice. The increased risk of intraoperative cyst rupture remains the main disadvantage for considering a laparoscopic approach. Intraoperative rupture may result in a theoretical risk of chemical peritonitis, spillage of malignant cells into the peritoneal cavity, and/or adhesion formation. Fortunately, many studies have failed to demonstrate any complications of chemical peritonitis following spillage of dermoid contents, supporting a minimally invasive approach [8]. Laparoscopic cystectomy is the preferred method of treating dermoid cysts, with the aim of preserving as much ovarian tissue as possible. Bilateral dermoids occur in 10 percent to 15 percent of cases; therefore, the contralateral ovary should always be visualized at the time of surgery. As the recurrence/persistence rate of dermoids following surgery is approximately 3 percent to 15 percent, follow-up with ultrasound 6–12 months postoperatively is recommended.

Adnexal Torsion

If torsion is suspected, prompt diagnosis and intervention are necessary to avoid long-term damage to the ovary and prevent oophorectomy. In cases of suspected ovarian torsion, detorsion with or without cystectomy has become the recommended surgical practice, even with a necrotic appearance of the ovary. Despite this recommendation, oophorectomy is still performed frequently at the time of ovarian torsion (30 percent to 86 percent).

Historically, it was recommended to remove the adnexa due to a theoretical risk that untwisting the ovarian pedicle would result in a thromboembolic event. Large retrospective series of detorsion have failed to demonstrate any patients with a thromboembolic event, further supporting a conservative surgical approach.

A laparoscopic approach is the preferred method of managing a presumed ovarian torsion. Usually, a three-port technique will suffice. The presence of a large ovarian mass (>8 cm) or suspected malignancy may preclude a laparoscopic approach but, fortunately, malignant lesions are particularly uncommon (<3 percent) in both the pediatric and adult populations.

Multiple studies have reported ovarian salvage following detorsion of the blue black ovary. Ovarian function has been documented at the time of follow-up ultrasound, following additional surgery, or following successful IVF [9].

Recurrence of torsion can result in an agonadal patient; therefore, prophylactic oophoropexy should be discussed at the time of surgery. The long-term effects of oophoropexy on fertility remain uncertain. Most surgeons consider performing this procedure when the ovarian ligament is congenitally long, in cases of repeat torsion, or when no obvious cause for the torsion is found. If an oophoropexy is carried out, the ovary is usually pexed to the pelvic side wall, back of the uterus, or the ipsilateral uterosacral ligament with either absorbable with nonabsorbable suture. Alternatively, the utero-ovarian ligament can be shortened [10] (Figure 11.1).

Endometriosis

The overall prevalence of endometriosis in adolescents with severe pelvic pain is very high (49 percent to 75 percent). The prevalence is higher in adolescents with chronic pelvic pain resistant to treatment

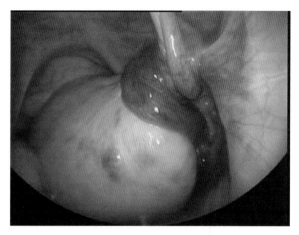

Figure 11.1 Photograph of an ovary with a cyst that has undergone torsion

compared to those who are responsive to treatment. Adolescents are often overlooked as their symptoms may be atypical and include non-cyclic pain, vague acute abdominal symptoms, gastrointestinal distress, and genitourinary symptoms. Sexually active teenagers may also report dyspareunia. Adolescents often have a delay in diagnosis of endometriosis from the onset of symptoms. The lack of noninvasive tools likely contributes to this delay. The goal of laparoscopic surgery is to make a diagnosis and to treat the bulk of disease conservatively in hopes of reducing pain and preserving fertility [11].

Usually, a three-port technique will suffice. Most adolescents (>60 percent) will have early-stage disease confined to the pelvis (Revised American Society for Reproductive medicine classification stage 1), but advanced endometriosis (stage 3 or 4) has been described, particularly in patients with early menstruation (<age 14) or obstructive anomalies. The risk of severe disease also appears to increase with advancing age.

It should be noted, however, that adolescent females with endometriosis often have subtle Atypical lesions that are clear, white, and red and not the powder-burn lesions commonly seen in adults. Familiarity with atypical lesions is paramount at the time of laparoscopy in making the correct diagnosis and treating active lesions [12]. A hydroflotation technique may help prevent collapse of the vascular network and filmy adhesions to allow for identification of these subtle lesions.

Treatment with either resection or ablation of endometriotic lesions and postoperative medical therapy has been shown to result in clinical improvement of endometriotic pain symptoms. Endometriosis surgery is cytoreductive rather than curative. An early diagnosis is believed by many authors to be an opportunity to intervene in the progressive nature of the disease. Unfortunately, the recurrence of pain and/or disease is a significant problem and appears to occur regardless of postoperative adjuvant therapy. It is not surprising that the need for a second surgery to treat recurrent symptoms has been reported to be as high as 34 percent 5 years postoperatively in an adolescent cohort. More recently, aggressive use of medical treatment and complementary/alternative therapies as first line for presumed and/or laparoscopically confirmed endometriosis has been suggested as a possible intervention to avoid surgery altogether. There is currently no consensus on whether this conservative approach is the correct one [13].

A major risk factor in severity of the endometriosis in the adolescent is a Mullerian anomaly resulting in an outflow obstruction. The incidence of endometriosis in this group of adolescents with genital tract anomalies varies between 6 percent and 40 percent. Surgical treatment of the outflow obstruction often will result in improvement of the disease or even spontaneous resolution, particularly if the disease was debulked at the initial surgery.

Gonadectomy, Vaginoplasty, and Complex Mullerian Anomalies

Gonadectomy

The investigations and timing of gonadectomy in girls with a 46XY disorder of sex development has been discussed elsewhere. In most situations, the surgery will be carried out in late adolescence, once puberty is complete. Two important factors need to be considered when undertaking the surgery: the first is to ensure complete excision of the gonads and the second is their preoperative localization. Due to the potential malignant transformation of any residual tissue, it is essential to ensure complete excision. Thus, it is recommended to remove the Fallopian tubes and to take both vascular pedicles a reasonable distance away from the gonadal tissue.

The gonad can lie in any position along the normal path of descent of a testis in the male. In addition, it may be streak in nature making identification difficult. Where the gonad lies in the inguinal canal, a urologist

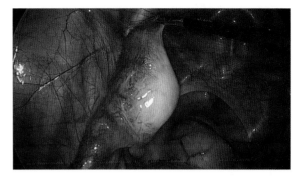

Figure 11.2 Gonads showing position higher in pelvis

will remove it through a groin incision. However, at times, with massage of the groin and pulling on the pedicle from the pelvic aspect, the gonad can be withdrawn back into the abdomen and removed laparoscopically. Conversely the gonad may lie higher up than expected and indeed outside the pelvis (Figure 11.2). Thus, the operation may be straightforward at times but on other occasions require dissection around the ureter or side-wall vessels.

Normally a three-port technique will suffice. A method to occlude the pedicle and then divide it is required. Technologies such as reusable bipolar and scissors may be employed, but more advanced energy sources that utilize ultrasonic make the surgery easier and more efficient. Where the pedicle is close to the ureter, the side wall may need to be opened and formal separation carried out to prevent ureteric injury due to heat spread. At the end of the procedure, it is preferable to remove the gonads separately: if the histology were to demonstrate malignant transformation, it is important to identify from which gonad it arose. Depending on whether or not a cyst was present on the gonad and hence the size, it may or may not be necessary to employ an extraction bag to remove the gonads from the abdomen.

Laparoscopic Creation of a Neovagina

The majority of women with a short blind-ending vagina (from conditions such as MRKH and CAIS) are able to use dilators with good effect. However, 20 percent will not get a satisfactory result or struggle with using dilators, especially if the perineum is flat with no vaginal dimple. These women can be offered a surgical procedure to create a functioning vagina. Most techniques were originally developed using laparotomy but are now performed laparoscopically.

145

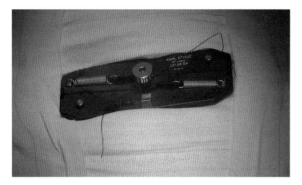

Figure 11.3 Picture of traction device used for a Vecchietti

Laparoscopic Vecchietti

Normally a three-port laparoscopy is used. The space between the bladder and rectum is opened so that a needle loaded with a suture can be passed into the pelvis from the vaginal dimple. A small acrylic olive is threaded and positioned in the vaginal dimple. The two ends of the thread are pulled from the vaginal dimple through the anterior abdominal wall and into a traction device (Figure 11.3). A cystoscopy is performed to exclude a bladder perforation during needle passing. The original description of this procedure suggests that the threads should be passed in a retroperitoneal fashion, but in our experience a trans-peritoneal path causes no problems. The device holds the threads under tension and, by turning a screw, shortens the threads evenly by 1 cm per day. This causes the olive to be pulled upward, creating an elongation of the vagina over a week; at that point, the traction device and beads are removed. The patient has a Foley catheter until the traction device is removed. Postoperative dilation and/or intercourse are required to maintain vaginal length [14].

Laparoscopic Davydov

In women who have no vaginal dimple or whose external genitalia are scarred (e.g., from perineal surgery around birth/infancy), a Davydov procedure can be performed. The space between the rectum and bladder is developed both from the perineum below and laparoscopically from above. The edges of the pelvic peritoneum are "pulled down" and attached to the dissected perineal skin with interrupted sutures to form a vagina lined with peritoneum. The open apex of the vagina is closed with an absorbable purse-string suture placed 11 to 13 cm from the opening of the neovagina. The peritoneum within the neovagina is replaced by squamous vaginal epithelium over the subsequent few months. This procedure would be difficult in patients who have undergone extensive abdominal surgery, as the peritoneum may not be sufficiently pliable to pull it down to the perineum.

Laparoscopic Intestinal Vaginoplasty

In patients who have previously had major abdominal surgery (such as bladder reconstruction for cloacal anomalies), intestinal vaginoplasty can be offered via a laparoscopic-assisted approach. A segment of bowel (usually sigmoid colon) is resected keeping its mesentery intact with one end of the bowel brought down to the perineum and sutured into place. Mucus production from the intestine can help with lubrication during intercourse; however, some women have to douche to get rid of excessive secretions.

Deciding Which Procedure to Use

Choosing which form of neovagina to offer depends on many factors and should only be considered if the woman is sufficiently motivated and psychologically ready. It makes sense to offer the least invasive procedure initially, so dilators should be offered before any surgical procedure is discussed. The choice of laparoscopic procedure will depend on history of previous surgery and the algorithm used by University College Hospital London aids the decision-making process (Figure 11.4).

Now that uterine transplantation has become a potential reality for women with uterine agenesis [15], the suitability of any neovagina to be connected to the transplanted cervix may need to be borne in mind in the future. Ideally, a simple neovagina made of skin, which does not have the rectum or bladder in close approximation to the vault would probably be the easiest to attach to a transplanted uterus.

Neovaginas formed using dilation or laparoscopically will lack apical support and so are at risk of prolapse. A vault prolapse occurring in this situation would normally be repaired using the same technique as in a sacrocolpopexy for post-hysterectomy vault prolapse. The risk of prolapse should be part of the counseling process before surgery.

Mullerian anomalies

Abnormal development of the Mullerian structures can lead to various structural anomalies, many of which need no treatment particularly if asymptomatic [16]. Anomalies that cause obstruction of menstrual flow such as a noncommunicating uterine horn, cervical agenesis, or transverse vaginal septa can present with

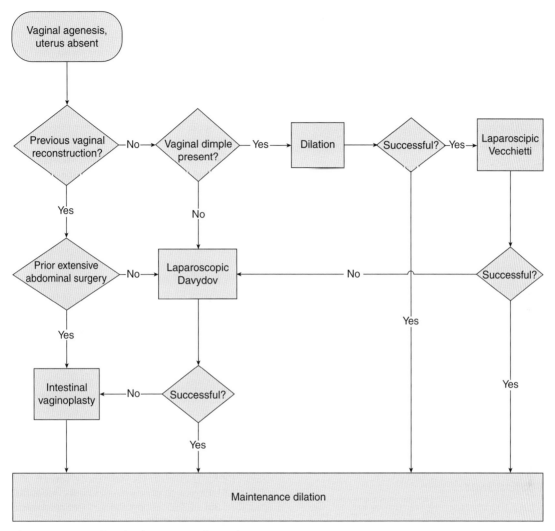

Figure 11.4 UCLH algorithm for treatment of vaginal agenesis

severe menstrual pain, or cyclical pain and primary amenorrhea if there is no normally communicating horn present.

Obstructed Uterine Horn

Treatment of an obstructed uterine horn (Figure 11.5) is by surgical excision of the horn. The attached Fallopian tube should also be removed to avoid the risk of an ectopic pregnancy from transperitoneal migration of sperm from the contralateral side where there is connection with the vagina. If the obstructed horn lies away from the functioning uterus, then the procedure is simple. However, if the horn is adjacent to the functioning uterus and covered by myometrium, then removal of the horn (and all of its endometrium and any

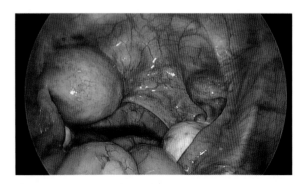

Figure 11.5 Photograph demonstrating two uterine horns. Small uterine horn on the right side wall and larger left-sided uterine horn.

147

rudimentary cervix) can be more challenging. The uterus can be extracted using mechanical morcellation. Preoperative imaging should ensure that the surgeon knows what to expect in terms of horn position and also the number of ureters and their location.

Women left with a unicornuate uterus should be warned that they are at increased risk of late miscarriage, preterm labor, and malpresentation/position in any subsequent pregnancy.

Cervical Agenesis

Historically cervical agenesis was treated by hysterectomy to solve the pain of obstructed menstruation. More recently, fertility-sparing surgery to perform a utero-vaginal anastomosis has been performed via laparotomy and laparoscopically [17]. The procedure involves a combined laparoscopic and perineal approach. From above, the bladder is reflected from the uterus, and a sound is introduced via the fundus to identify the level of obstruction. The distal end of the obstruction is canalized from the perineum with a combination of sharp and blunt dissection. The fibromuscular tissue at the level of the obstruction is then resected and the distal uterus connected to the upper vagina in a combined laparoscopic and perineal approach. A Foley catheter is left (deflated) in the uterine cavity extending into the vagina to prevent stenosis of the new canal, which is removed under anesthetic about 1 month later.

Transverse Vaginal Septa

In cases where the obstructing septum is low in the vagina, excision is performed via a vaginal approach. In cases of high vagina septum, a combined abdominoperineal approach must be utilized.

If the vagina and uterus are very distended, then a Palmer's point entry is advisable. The utero-vesical peritoneum is opened and the bladder reflected down. The anterior aspect of the distended obstructed vagina is opened transversely and the hematocolpos drained. The transverse vaginal septum can then be excised and the incision enlarged from below using Hegar dilators. A device such as a McCartney tube can then be used to maintain the pneumoperitoneum. The proximal and distal vaginas can then be anastomosed using interrupted absorbable sutures. This can either be performed vaginally or laparoscopically depending on the vaginal access. The anterior vaginal defect is then sutured laparoscopically. A vaginal pack and catheter are left in situ overnight [18].

References

1. Medeiros LRF, Rosa DD, Bozzetti MC, Fachel JMG, Furness S, Garry R et al. Laparoscopy versus laparotomy for benign ovarian tumour. Cochrane Database of Systematic Reviews 2009, Issue 2. Art. No.: CD004751. DOI: 10.1002/14651858.CD004751.pub3.

2. Cutner A. Stavroulis A. Zolfaghari N. Risk assessment of the ergonomic aspects of laparoscopic theatre. *Gynecol Surg.* 2013; **10**(2): 99–102.

3. Stravroulis A, Cutner A, Liao L-M. Staff perceptions of the effects of an integrated laparoscopic theatre environment on teamwork. *Gynecol Surg* 2013; **10**(3): 177–80.

4. Royal College of Obstetricians and Gynecologists. Preventing entry-related gynecological laparoscopic injuries. Green-top guideline number 49. London, RCOG. www.rcog.org.uk/en/guidelines-research -services/guidelines/gtg49/.

5. Aust TR, Kayani SI, Rowlands DJ. Direct optical entry through Palmer's point; a new technique for those at risk of entry-related trauma at laparoscopy. *Gynecol Surg.* 2010; **7**(3): 315–17.

6. Brandner B, Krishnan P, Sitham M, Man A, Saridogan E, Cutner A. Is naso-gastric tube insertion necessary to reduce the risk of gastric injury at subcostal laparoscopic insufflation? A pilot study. *Eur J Anaesthesiol.* 2007; **24**(7): 644–45.

7. Cutner AS, Lazanakis MS, Saridogan E. Laparoscopic ovarian suspension to facilitate surgery for advanced endometriosis. *Fertil Steril.* 2004; **82**(3): 702–4.

8. Savasi I, Lacy JA, Gerstle JT, Stephens D, Kives S, Allen L. Management of ovarian dermoid cysts in the pediatric and adolescent population. *J Pediatr Adolesc Gynecol.* 2009; **22**(6): 360–64.

9. Oelsner G, Cohen SB, Soriano D, Admon D, Mashiach S, Carp H. Minimal surgery for the twisted ischaemic adnexa can preserve ovarian function. *Hum Reprod.* 2003; **18**(12): 2599–602.

10. Rossi BV, Ference EH, Zurakowski D, Scholz S, Feins NR, Chow JS, Laufer MR. The clinical presentation and surgical management of adnexal torsion in the pediatric and adolescent population. *J Pediatr Adolesc Gynecol.* 2012; **25**(2): 109–13.

11. Brosens I, Gordts S, Benagiano G. Endometriosis in adolescents is a hidden, progressive and severe disease that deserves attention, not just compassion. *Hum Reprod.* 2013; **28**(8): 2026–31.

12. Dun EC, Kho KA, Morozov VV, Kearney S, Zurawin JL, Nezhat CH. Endometriosis in adolescents. *JSLS.* 2015; **19**(2).

13. Sarıdoğan E. Adolescent endometriosis. *Eur J Obstet Gynecol Reprod Biol.* 2016; **209**: 46–49.

14. Ismail I, Cutner A, Creighton S. Laparoscopic vaginoplasty: alternative techniques in vaginal reconstruction. *BJOG: An International Journal of Obstetrics & Gynecology*, 2006; **113**: 340–43.

15. Brännström M, Johannesson L, Bokström H, Kvarnström N, Mölne J, Dahm-Kähler P et al. Livebirth after uterus transplantation. *Lancet*. 2015; **385**(9968): 607–16.

16. Vallerie AM, Breech LL. Update in Mullerian anomalies: diagnosis, management, and outcomes. *Curr Opin Obstet Gynecol*. 2010; **22**(5): 381–87.

17. Creighton SM, Davies MC, Cutner A. Laparoscopic management of cervical agenesis. *Fertil Steril*. 2006; **85**(5): 1510.

18. Williams CE, Cutner AC, Creighton SM. Laparoscopic management of high transverse vaginal septae: a case report. *Gynecol Surg*. 2013; **10**(3): 189–191.

Chapter 12

Psychological Care in Pediatric and Adolescent Gynecology Practice: Addressing the Effects of Sexual and Gender Norms

Julie Alderson, Katrina Roen, and Miriam Muscarella

We offer the chapter with a list of practical suggestions for adopting a norm-critical approach in providing health care for girls and women (Table 12.1).

In acute hospitals in the UK, health care psychologists work within specialist health care teams including pediatric and adolescent gynecology (PAG) services. Their role with patients is to maximize function and minimize distress associated with chronic physical health conditions. In PAG, the conditions may include menstrual problems, differences of sex development, gynecological cancer, and pelvic or genital pain.

Re-engagement with preferred life goals and maintenance of relationships following body-altering illness or treatment are a typical clinical focus for psychologists. Women who have experienced genital trauma or birth complications or have been sexually abused may require psychological therapy to enable them to undergo essential medical investigations and treatment. Psychological interventions can also boost the effectiveness of medical treatments via motivational and behavior-change strategies to improve adherence to self-management.

These activities, tackle health, illness, and health care experiences at an individual and familial level. Psychological research and practice in health care has been criticized for its weak conceptualization of societal framing of human experiences [1,2]. At the simplest level, a care provider and care recipient transaction is a meeting between two social beings, typically in an unequal relationship. At another level, there is a subtle collision of two sets of perceptions, assumptions, expectations, and values. One such set of perceptions concerns social norms, that is, our preconceived

ideas of what is socially acceptable. *Critical* psychologists (psychologists who challenge mainstream approaches) consider it imperative for care providers to be alive to the values (and value judgments) that are shaping thought and action in doctor-patient interaction and health care processes overall.

This chapter focuses on medical conditions that challenge social norms for bodily appearance and function and sexual practices. We present arguments for positioning multi-professional care for affected girls and women within a norm-critical framework. While we recognize the impact of social pressure to achieve normalcy via medical interventions, we present alternative approaches that respect diversity in body and identity and encourage PAG specialists to question conformity to gendered norms as a treatment goal. In the final section, we present the clinical management of vaginal agenesis as an example of how to offer the service differently, These principles are applicable to a range of PAG conditions including vulval appearance distress, vulvodynia, pelvic pain, or ovarian failure.

Normative Pressure

Research into sex differences, gender identity (identifying as a woman or man), and sexuality (partner choice, fantasy, activity) has continued apace since medical researchers began to focus on psychosexual development [3]. However, health professionals typically aim to modify, restore, or repair toward "normal" function, as if "functions" relating to gender and sexuality are straightforward entities. It has been argued that normal femininity and masculinity are constructed and contested realities that cannot be reliably defined [3]. In devising treatment plans, it is important to be aware of the values and assumptions embedded in the goal of treatment.

We thank dsdfamilies.org for the permission to reproduce pages 18 and 19 of Ten Top Tips for Dilation and Lih-Mei Liao for the editorial suggestions and improvements to the manuscript.

Table 12.1 List of strategies for a norm-critical approach in PAG

1. Assure families that they cannot alter their child's gender identity or sexual orientation.
2. Allow the family and patient to be norm-critical and question:

    Are we feeling pressure to be "normal" (a normal girl, woman, female) and what do we actually want for our child/ourselves?

3. Use early conversations with parents to build positive body understandings and help them find language they can use with their child.
4. Take time to discuss the body with the young person without emphasizing deficiency or pathology, and consider using peer-oriented approaches to develop body understanding.
5. Elicit the young person's understandings of her body, including what interests her as well as what concerns her about her body.
6. Beware of over-examining and consider patient-centered approaches to determining whether and when examinations are needed.
7. Approach conversations about options in care with an emphasis on the girl's or young woman's own role in deciding what is right for her, and when.
8. Ensure that some conversations happen without the parents in the room, and review conversations or decisions that have been led by parents.
9. Integrate self-discovery and pleasure into processes that might otherwise be medicalized, such as dilatation, allowing the patient to determine which method works for her.
10. Explicitly provide opportunities for the patient to change her mind without any negative repercussions.

Many individuals, families, and communities may have a more flexible perspective on sex and gender than health professionals. Fluidity in gendered identification and behavior in childhood is arguably more acceptable for families and communities than is assumed by clinicians and researchers. For example, research in the relationship between prenatal hormones and gendered behavior in girls with classical congenital adrenal hyperplasia (CAH) rarely draws attention to the fact that these effects are not necessarily considered a problem by the children and their families [4]. Attitudes in the wider culture, which may be reflected in the family or the health professional's behaviors, will affect the children's *interpretation* of their gender development and influence their self-acceptance and self-esteem.

Because the development of gender identity and sexuality continues across the lifespan, medical interventions in childhood and adolescence can have unknown consequences. Norm-critical approaches offer a way of thinking about questions often taken for granted, such as What is *normal*? What does

it mean to be a *woman*? What kinds of bodies can be called *female*? From a norm-critical perspective, it is assumed that not all girls will grow up to be women. Some girls will become transmen, who may or may not retain their female-typical anatomy. Furthermore, it is important to recognize that not all young women seek sexual relationships with men, not all heterosexual women seek to engage in coitus, and many people do not aspire to a typical sex anatomy [5].

In clinical consultations, patients react to verbal and nonverbal cues that may inhibit or encourage their own expressions and, importantly, how they should decide. Without the capacity to reflect on practice, clinicians may subtly steer their patients toward conformity to social expectations in sex and gender that lead to fear and shame for some individuals. Likewise, how a genital examination is conducted might indicate to the patient that her body is worrying.

☒	☑
Discussing elective interventions for a woman with CAH:	
"Would you like to be referred to a voice trainer to feminize your voice?"	*"Please tell us about any concerns that you may have about living with CAH."*
This presumes that the patient wants to conform to gender norms.	This allows the patient to name her own concerns without preempting them.

Without the conscious intention to reflect on language and practice, the clinician may inadvertently privilege some patients and disadvantage others. For example, in routinely introducing fertility options, the clinician is assuming that all women want to become mothers. This may valorize the wish to become mothers and diminish women who up until this point have felt disinclined toward motherhood.

☒	☑
After identifying a fertility challenge:	
"You can still have children; these are your options …"	*"Some people want to be parents and some don't. We can discuss the options if and when, or not at all."*
This suggests to the patient that she should be interested in becoming a mother.	This opens up the topic of parenting without communicating any right or wrong in how the patient chooses.

Some clinicians may unknowingly silence patients who do not conform to social norms or feel uncomfortable discussing them. Others may be too eager to help women yield to normative pressure, such as removing healthy and sensuous labial tissue of girls and women. It is important to be wary of the misappropriation of patient "choice" when such "choice" is a manifestation of oppressive cultural values for women [6]. Interventions to meet social expectations may be doomed to fail, as idealized genitalia are not surgically altered genitalia [7,8].

Accepting Diversity

To consider the bodies of girls and women as diverse and functioning differently is to recognize the possibilities for fulfillment of their potential. Clinicians, parents, and individuals might usefully think about how the body can function as it is and what adaptations in behavior, attitude, or expectation can optimize function.

Communicating with Parents

Raising resilient children who competently manage health and development issues rests heavily on parenting. The style of communication between parents and health professionals, following the diagnosis of a childhood condition, makes a significant difference in parents' ability to understand the medical process ahead and to foster their child's well-being through that process [9,10]. Focusing primarily on intervention and modification at this stage suggests there is a need to "right a wrong." This is far from helpful when communicating with parents about the day-to-day problems that they and their child may face.

✖	✔
Reaching a diagnosis and planning care with parents:	
"Now we have a diagnosis, we will introduce you to our surgeons and psychologist to talk about treatment."	*"Now that we know more about you and your baby, let's discuss how our team can support you all now and in the future"*
This presumes that treatment is a priority for the service and immediately puts parents under pressure.	This ensures that the welfare of the baby and family is the central focus of the service

Consultations with parents concerning an infant who is different can be highly emotional, and the medical information that resonates with parental emotions is more likely to be remembered. How a condition is explained forms the basis of the parents' narratives about their child [11]. Extreme emotions can prevent parents from having a thorough discussion about their child's care plan and making clear-headed decisions as discussed in chapter 5. Parents should therefore be encouraged to take notes and be given information leaflets to keep for later, for example, when explaining their decision to the child. Ideally their relationship with the multidisciplinary team (MDT) will enable parents to express concerns, seek specific information, and be open to thinking about normative pressure that may be influencing them.

Privacy without Shame

Parents' primary aims for their children typically include happiness and self-worth. This often includes a wish that their child will love and be loved. Because relationships with the primary caregivers are a training ground for loving and caring relationships throughout life, many parents know that the child and her body should be respected and cherished by them, and by the child. This tacit knowledge of the importance of a positive relationship with one's body, no matter how unwell or atypical it is, can sit confusingly alongside concerns about teasing or stigma. Parents whose child is "different" in any way may be concerned for the child, and may feel highly anxious. Clinical consultations can support parents in finding ways to show their child that she and her body is acceptable and lovable, as well as providing strategies for reducing parental anticipatory anxiety. These can involve working out with parents some practical things they can do with their child including cognitive-behavioural strategies.

It is useful to discuss the difference between privacy (teaching the child that she has the right to share aspects of her body with trusted persons) versus secrecy (teaching the child that her medical condition must be kept secret). Emphasizing secrecy can foster shame and anxiety in the person concerned [12]. It is important to ascertain whether the parents believe that the child's difference must be kept secret. If parents have negative feelings about their child's diagnosis and believe that information must be withheld from the child, direct psychological intervention can be helpful.

☒	☑
Talking about diverse bodies:	
"You must talk to your child about her diagnosis. She can still be discrete about her private parts and the fact that she can't carry a baby. She can tell it all to the special person when she is in a trusting relationship."	*"Learning about how everyone's body is different and about how bodies work are important aspects of growing up for all of us. The conversations you and your child have about this will help her know that she is loved and her body is loveable."*
This could be understood to emphasize secrecy (and, implicitly, shame) rather than learning, self-discovery, and pleasure.	This emphasizes supporting the child to get to know and appreciate her own body and accept human diversity.

Young People at the Center of Care

It is understood as standard practice that children and young people are to be told in age-appropriate ways about any diagnosis and treatment [13] and involved in decision making when possible [14]. However, there is usually a gap between theory and action. Many clinicians consider it the parents' responsibility to talk with their child, even though some parents feel unable or are unwilling to do this [15]. A primary aim of the PAG team, then, is to assist the parents to help the child understand her body. To do this in a way that encourages the child to accept and cherish her body, information should be presented to the child using materials and terms that are free from associations with illness and medical intervention. From this general understanding of the human body, it may then be possible to talk about the child's own body, that is, what she needs to learn about her body, how she wants to experience her body, and how she intends to talk to others about her body or not. Finally, the talk can move toward health care interventions: what is offered, and why, and what are the experiences of others who have (or have not) had the proposed interventions. The young person should be supported to think about and express how she feels about her body and the interventions offered. The conversations should champion diversity and difference. There is a vital role here for partnership working with voluntary agencies and care user groups.

☒	☑
Centralizing the person and her body rather than the treatment:	
"Before your examination under anesthesia we will make sure you understand what we want to look at, and we can talk about the treatment plan."	*"If you can understand more about how your body works, it will help you think about what kind of medical care you might want from us in the future."*
This puts medical intervention first, and does not consider the way a person experiences their own body.	This puts the person's own experience first and signals that medical interventions are secondary and not (necessarily) needed.

When a child or young person requires medical investigations and interventions without delay, such as in cases of hematacolpos, there is a risk of suboptimal information sharing. Nevertheless, the child or young person must be the primary and active contributor within her care. Even within short time scales, she should be given time with a member of the MDT when she can express what she understands and demonstrate how she could (or does) talk with friends, family, and possibly others. A silent child may not have understood what is being said. This can be a challenging aspect of working with children since passivity is often culturally synonymous with being a "good" patient. Parents may need our help to engage the child. Non-life-saving treatment including puberty induction should not be undertaken without the child's good enough understanding of the implications.

Body Image

Adolescence can be a time of increased pressure to conform to social norms, particularly in relation to sexed appearance and sexual interactions. Psychological support for children and young people can usefully include work on the topics of bodily norms (what ordinary bodies really look like and how they work) and normative pressure (building a critical awareness of societal pressure to conform). A person whose genital appearance or function has been affected by a medical condition, or whose sex development is not typical, should ideally be prepared for, and supported through, the challenges of adolescence and changing peer relationships. The MDT and parents should be able to talk about the fact that bodies develop in diverse ways and everybody deviates from perceived norms in some way. There should be opportunities for the young person to develop an understanding of how normative pressure operates, and strategies for dealing with the pressures that may arise in their lives. Psychological work can be particularly important when a young person is comparing her body with peers' bodies and finding the differences to be overwhelmingly distressing. For some, this plays into a fantasy that medical intervention will make the psychological effects of normative pressure disappear.

☒	☑
Resisting normative pressure and appreciating diverse bodies:	
"There are different treatments to make the vagina bigger so you can have sex."	*"People make such different choices about how they explore sexual feelings and activities, by themselves or with a partner. We are here to support your choices as and when you are ready."*
This presumes that the person wants to have a vagina of a particular size and conflates sex with coitus.	This acknowledges the diversity of sexual expressions and avoids medicalizing the patient's sexuality.

Body image problems involve three main components in an individual's reaction to her physical being: affective (e.g., shame, unease, dissatisfaction, unhappiness), cognitive (e.g., discontent, desire for change), and behavioral (e.g., avoidance, concealment). In relation to PAG conditions, body image relates to how a girl or young woman feels about her body as sexed, as sexually desirable and desiring, and how she feels about her body in sexual interaction with others. Girls and young women who face particular difficulties may believe that they and their bodies are unlovable. Some may avoid intimacy altogether. They may picture for themselves a future that is devoid of romantic relationships and sexual intimacy.

Repeated exposure to physical examination may lead to the individual adopting the observer's perspective on her body. Concerns about the impact is reflected in recent guidelines that urge against the overuse of gynecological examinations [16]. Over-examination might mean that a young person comes to consider her sexual anatomy as something outside her own control and not in terms of pleasure. Self-objectification has been identified as contributing to body image problems. Issues of bodily self-consciousness and sexual esteem, that is, the value that one places on oneself as a sexual being [17], can also impact on sexual function. Here, in considering concepts such as objectification and sexual esteem, we are drawing attention to the cognitive aspects of body image. These can include dissociation (feeling cutoff) from the physical sensations and emotions of sexual intimacy [18].

The way that people perceive and feel about their bodies is also affected by what they learn about others' bodies. Popular beliefs about the uniformity of female genitalia persist despite clinically established knowledge about variation in appearance of the postpubertal vulva [19]. Given that positive genital perceptions have been linked to increased sexual esteem and lower distress during sexual intimacy, it is worth undertaking preventative psychological work to mitigate risks associated with genital dissatisfaction. In PAG, this can involve supporting parents to raise their children in line with an approach that promotes talking about sex development, bodily norms, and bodily difference. This will help a young person develop a language for her experience as her sexuality develops. Ideally, the language developed will enable the young person to make decisions about her body, to seek information about medical interventions, and to seek others with similar conditions and experiences. A young person could usefully become familiar with medicalized terms, as well as popular and age-appropriate terms that are non-stigmatizing.

☒	☑
Explaining diverse and typical body function:	
"Having CAH means your clitoris is bigger than usual. You might experience clitoral erections when you are aroused or with your boyfriend. This is entirely normal and not a worry."	*"All bodies are different. When people are sexually aroused or turned on, the genitals can feel fuller and more sensitive, and this is true of the clitoris. You might notice this when you feel turned on."*
This emphasizes clitoral size. The word "erection" may be shaming. It presumes that the person is heterosexual and has (or will have) a boyfriend. It precludes autoerotic activities in which she may engage.	*"For some people, the clitoris is more hidden. For others it is more visible. Whether more hidden or visible, the clitoris can become fuller and more sensitive when the person is aroused."*
	This places genital differences on a spectrum of human diversity. It refers to sexual arousal using popular terminology, and it refers to genital engorgement in language that suggests something pleasurable and non-stigmatizing.

As the young person reaches an age when she might talk about sexual relationships, it will be necessary to provide consultation time with the appropriate MDT member, without the presence of a parent. Discussing a range of sexual practices, experiences, and sensations that may be part of a sexual relationship helps introduce and validate diverse sexualities. For young women who have had genital surgery earlier in their lives, it may be particularly relevant to talk about genital sensation and appearance. It can be extremely anxiety provoking to allow another person to see or touch one's genitals during a sexual encounter when the prior genital contact has been in a medical setting. Working sensitively with young people can help them prepare for embarking on intimacy with resilience and in ways that are less likely to result in rejection.

When interventions such as puberty induction, vagina dilation, and gonadectomy are offered to young people, tailored education, taking into account emerging debates in the literature, is needed to help the young person make an informed choice. Without this, a young person who is embarrassed about her difference, or has difficulty seeing herself as a sexual being, or has confused feelings about fertility may become passive in relation to the medical team. She could hear an *offer* of treatment as a statement that her body needs to be altered to be acceptable. It is important to begin discussions from the understanding that diverse sexual appearance and function are acceptable, do not always need alteration, and will not necessarily impede sexual enjoyment or relationships. While diverse or "different" bodies do not impair sexual relationships, experiences of stigma, fear, and shame about one's body do. Clinicians have a duty of care to avoid being a source of social pressure as they discuss elective medical interventions with their patients.

☒	☑
Offering elective procedures:	
"A short or dimple vagina responds well to dilation treatment in MRKH, enabling you to have sex."	*"Many women want to have intercourse, many others don't. Women who have not developed with a vagina sometimes choose dilation to prepare for sexual intercourse. This can work well for some people and not others. It is a choice."*

(cont.)

☒	☑
This implicitly states that the only way to have sex is via penetration. It places the diagnosis and treatment at the center, rather than focusing on the woman and her own experience of her body.	This validates a range of sexual activities and indicates that penetrative sex is only one possibility and is not a necessity. It makes it clear that dilation is elective.

An Example of Norm-Critical Care: Vaginal Agenesis

Research into the holistic care for women with vaginal agenesis is lacking. Thus far, the focus has been on producing a vagina of a particular size rather than sexual experience. In prioritizing genital intercourse as a goal of treatment, the male partner's satisfaction is privileged over and above the woman's pleasure. Multidisciplinary care should begin with the tacit understanding that the woman's experience of her body and her sexual pleasure are the primary outcomes, and that vagina construction is not a prerequisite for positive sexual experiences and treatment has a potentially negative impact on sexual experience.

Treatment for a woman who does not have a vaginal opening, or whose vagina is shorter or narrower than typical, often begins with a daily self-managed dilation regime that lasts several months. Knowledge, skills, and motivation are central to adherence to such a demanding regime and can be enhanced with specialist psychological input. The demanding task of dilation may also require a clarity of purpose that is part of the individual's emotional maturity. Possible emotional barriers or complications may include memories of abuse or a history of sexual rejection. The process of assessment of readiness, preparation, and support should be thorough.

Given that there are different routes to stretching vaginal width or length, the patient should be encouraged to prioritize her own goals and psychological comfort throughout this challenging process. The approach may be introduced to the patient as being on a continuum from a mostly medicalized to a mostly pleasure-oriented approach. A medicalized approach could be characterized by an instruction such as "Use the dilator for 20–30 minutes at the scheduled times." A pleasure-oriented approach might involve a suggestion such as "Experiment with a vibrator (for penetration) while masturbating

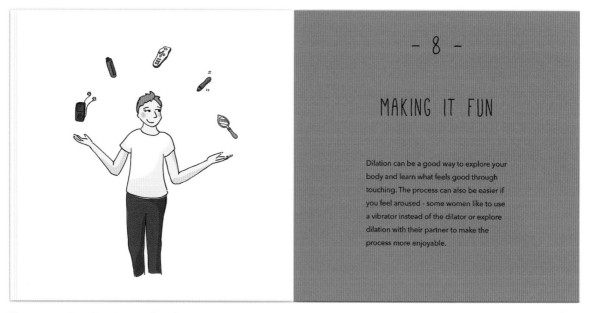

– 8 –

MAKING IT FUN

Dilation can be a good way to explore your body and learn what feels good through touching. The process can also be easier if you feel aroused - some women like to use a vibrator instead of the dilator or explore dilation with their partner to make the process more enjoyable.

Figure 12.1 From "Top Ten Tips for Dilation," reproduced with the permission of dsdfamilies.org

or love making so that once aroused you might experience the pressure as pleasurable." A mixture of ideas guided by the patient's wishes is best. Supporting resources that appeal to the patient are helpful. Furthermore, the service must be willing to modify the approach and timing.

A team member able to discuss psychosexual matters openly is a great asset to the service. He or she can help the team shift the treatment goal from normalizing anatomy to encouraging women to prioritize pleasure and intimacy in sexual activities. This input may involve information not widely available in clinical settings such as the alternative or additional use of vibrators, erotic media, lubricants, as well as practical advice such as warming dilators, increasing frequency of use, involving a partner, talking with others going through the process, finding privacy, and using deep breathing to aid the process. Tools such as the "Top Ten Tips for Dilation" produced by a user group in collaboration with psychologists, gynecologists, and artists [20] (Figure 12.1) may serve as a starting place. A person-centered or individualized approach to dilator use can help with the transition from clinical touch to erotic touch and may reduce the potential negative effects of objectification of the patient's genitals. Assuring patients that dilation is also for women with typical sex anatomies may help.

Conclusions

The pressure to regulate bodily appearance and function and sexual practices to meet social expectations can lead patients and professionals down a difficult path characterized by confusion, dilemma, and dissatisfaction. With a greater awareness of the powerful influence of normative pressure on clinical practice, PAG specialists can begin to move away from the over-focus on normalcy to put the welfare of girls and women at the heart of their practice. PAG specialists who are able to adjust their professional values in such a way stand to have a profoundly positive impact on young people's self-worth and sexual wellness.

References

1. Suls J, Wallston KA. (Eds.). *Social Psychological Foundations of Health and Illness.* Oxford, UK: Wiley-Blackwell 2003.

2. Ussher JM. Reproductive rhetoric and the blaming of the body. In P Nicholson, JM Ussher (Eds.). *The Psychology of Women's Health and Healthcare.* London: Macmillan 2002, pp. 31–61.

3. Liao L. Development of sexuality: psychological perspectives. In A Balen, S Creighton, M Davies, J MacDougall, R Stanhope (Eds.). *Pediatric and Adolescent Gynaecology: A Multidisciplinary Approach.* Cambridge: Cambridge University Press 2004, pp. 77–93.

4. Pasterski V, Zucker KJ, Hindmarsh PC, Hughes IA, Acerini C, Spencer D. et al. Increased cross-gender identification independent of gender role behaviour in girls with congenital adrenal hyperplasia: results from a standardized assessment of 4- to 11-year-old children. *Archives of Sexual Behavior* 2015; **44**: 136–37. doi:10.1007/s10508-014-0385-0

5. Clarke V, Peel E. *Out in Psychology: Lesbian, Gay, Bisexual, Trans and Queer Perspectives*. Chichester, West Sussex, England; Hoboken, NJ: John Wiley & Sons 2007.

6. Lippman A. Choice as a risk to women's health. *Health, Risk & Society* 1999; **1**(3): 281–91. doi:10.1080/13698579908406317

7. Holmes M. Queer cut bodies. In JAD Boone, M Meeker, K Quimby, C Sarver, D Silverman, -R Weatherston (Eds.). *Queer Frontiers: Millennial Geographies, Genders, and Generations*. Madison: University of Wisconsin Press 2002, pp. 84–110.

8. Roen K. "But we have to do something": Surgical "correction" of atypical genitalia. *Body & Society* 2008; **14**(1): 4766.

9. Lundberg T, Lindström A, Roen K, Hegarty P. From knowing nothing to knowing now: Parents' experiences of caring for their children with Congenital Adrenal Hyperplasia. *Journal of Pediatric Psychology* 2016; 1–10. doi:10.1093/jpepsy/jsw001

10. Sanders C, Carter B, Goodacre L. Parents need to protect: influences, risks and tensions for parents of prepubertal children born with ambiguous genitalia. *Journal of Clinical Nursing* 2012; **21**(21–22): 3315.

11. Gough B, Weyman N, Alderson J, Butler G, Stoner M. "They did not have a word": The parental quest to locate a "true sex" for their intersex children. *Psychology & Health* 2008; **23**(4): 493–507. doi:10.1080/14768320601176170

12. Keenan KF, van Teijlingen E, McKee L, Miedzybrodzka Z, Simpson SA. How young people find out about their family history of Huntington's disease. *Social Science & Medicine* 2009; **68**(10): 1892–900. doi:10.1016/j.socscimed.2009.02.049

13. Vaknin O, Zisk-Rony RY. Including children in medical decisions and treatments: perceptions and practices of healthcare providers. *Child: Care, Health and Development* 2011; **37**(4): 533–39. doi:10.1111/j.1365-2214.2010.01153.x

14. Carmichael P, Alderson J. Psychological care in disorders of sexual differentiation and determination. In Adam Balen et al (Eds.). *Pediatric and adolescent gynaecology*. Cambridge: Cambridge University Press 2004, pp. 158–78.

15. Carmichael P, Ransley PG. Telling children about a physical intersex condition. *Dialogues in Pediatric Urology* (2002); **25**(6): 7–8.

16. Qaseem A, Humphrey LL, Harris R, Starkey M, Denberg TD. Screening pelvic examination in adult women: a clinical practice guideline from the American College of Physicians screening pelvic examination in adult women. *Annals of Internal Medicine* 2014; **161**(1): 67–72. doi:10.7326/M14-0701

17. Mayers, KS, Heller, DK Heller, JA Damaged Self-Esteem: A Kind of Disability. *Sexuality and Disability* 2003; **21**: 269.

18. O'Sullivan LF, Meyer-Bahlburg HFL, McKeague IW. The development of the sexual self-concept inventory for early adolescent girls. *Psychology of Women Quarterly* 2006; **30**(2): 139–49.

19. Lloyd J, Crouch NS, Minto CL, Liao L-M, Creighton SM. Female genital appearance: "normality" unfolds. *BJOG: An International Journal of Obstetrics and Gynaecology* 2015; **112**(5): 643–46.

20. Dsdfamilies. Top Ten Tips for Dilation. Retrieved from dsdfamilies.org, September 2016.

Index